A Comprehensive Textbook of

Psoriasis

A Comprehensive Textbook of Psoriasis

Peerzada Sajad Ahmad MD
Registrar
Department of Dermatology
Sexually Transmitted Disease (STD) and Leprosy
Government Medical College (GMC)
Srinagar, Jammu and Kashmir, India

Iffat Hassan MD
Professor and Head
Department of Dermatology
Sexually Transmitted Disease (STD) and Leprosy
Government Medical College (GMC)
Srinagar, Jammu and Kashmir, India

JAYPEE The Health Sciences Publisher
New Delhi | London | Philadelphia | Panama

Jaypee Brothers Medical Publishers (P) Ltd

Headquarters
Jaypee Brothers Medical Publishers (P) Ltd
4838/24, Ansari Road, Daryaganj
New Delhi 110 002, India
Phone: +91-11-43574357
Fax: +91-11-43574314
Email: jaypee@jaypeebrothers.com

Overseas Offices

J.P. Medical Ltd
83 Victoria Street, London
SW1H 0HW (UK)
Phone: +44 20 3170 8910
Fax: +44 (0)20 3008 6180
Email: info@jpmedpub.com

Jaypee-Highlights Medical Publishers Inc.
City of Knowledge, Bld. 235, 2nd Floor, Clayton
Panama City, Panama
Phone: +1 507-301-0496
Fax: +1 507-301-0499
Email: cservice@jphmedical.com

Jaypee Medical Inc.
325 Chestnut Street
111 South Independence Mall East
Suite 412, Philadelphia, PA 19106, USA
Phone: +1 267-519-9789
Email: support@jpmedus.com

Jaypee Brothers Medical Publishers (P) Ltd
17/1-B Babar Road, Block-B, Shaymali
Mohammadpur, Dhaka-1207
Bangladesh
Mobile: +08801912003485
Email: jaypeedhaka@gmail.com

Jaypee Brothers Medical Publishers (P) Ltd
Bhotahity, Kathmandu, Nepal
Phone: +977-9741283608
Email: kathmandu@jaypeebrothers.com

Website: www.jaypeebrothers.com
Website: www.jaypeedigital.com

Inquiries for bulk sales may be solicited at: jaypee@jaypeebrothers.com

A Comprehensive Textbook of Psoriasis

First Edition: **2016**

ISBN: 978-93-85999-82-6

Printed at Sanat Printers

Dedicated to

Our parents, family, friends and teachers

PREFACE

Being a student of dermatology and having gone through the difficult phase of residency, I know the demands and expectations of teachers and the traumatic phase the residents of dermatology go through their period of residency. Psoriasis as we all know is a disease which is characterized by remissions and relapses and is associated with considerable psychosocial morbidity, and every teacher wants his/her students to know everything about psoriasis because of the daily encounter with the disease, be it either in out-patient or in-patient department. Although there are a number of excellent textbooks available on the subject of psoriasis, but none of these have focused on all the issues related to the disease. In this textbook we have made an attempt to look at almost all the aspects of psoriasis, and I am pretty much sure that it will help the students to know psoriasis in depth and prepare for the examinations as well. Recent burning issues in psoriasis, such as metabolic syndrome, psychosocial morbidity, childhood psoriasis, biologicals in psoriasis and non-pharmacological treatments are a special feature of this textbook. I strongly believe that it will be of immense help to the students and teachers alike.

Suggestions and criticism from the readers are welcome.

Peerzada Sajad Ahmad

Dermatology as a subject has seen a sea change in the past few decades, with extensive research and consequently there has been a change in the aptitude of teaching, research and professional practice as well. Psoriasis as we all know is a disease which is characterized by remissions and relapses and give patients a lot of psychological stress. Although there are a handful of excellent textbooks available on the subject of psoriasis, but, all the aspects of psoriasis have not been addressed in those textbooks, hence a need was felt to contribute to the existing knowledge of psoriasis by writing a textbook with an attempt to focus on almost all aspects of the disease process. An attempt has been made to write it in a simple and lucid manner so that it can serve as a ready reckoner to postgraduates and those practicing dermatology. Recent burning issues in psoriasis, such as metabolic syndrome, psychosocial morbidity, childhood psoriasis, biologicals in psoriasis and non-pharmacological treatments are a special feature of this textbook. I believe it will be of immense help to the students and teachers alike.

Iffat Hassan

ACKNOWLEDGMENTS

The present work would not have been possible without the contribution and continuous encouraging support of several of our colleagues; Dr Imran Majid (Associate Professor, Department of Dermatology, GMC, Srinagar), Dr Yasmeen Jabeen (Assistant Professor, Department of Dermatology, GMC, Srinagar), Dr Shagufta Rather (Assistant Professor, Department of Dermatology, GMC, Srinagar) and Dr Syed Mubashir (Lecturer, Department of Dermatology, GMC, Srinagar); senior residents (Dr Gousia Sheikh, Dr Atiya Yaseen, Dr Abid Keen and Dr Safiya Bashir); and postgraduates (Dr Sumaya Zeerak, Dr Insha Latif, Dr Waseem, Dr Shazmeen, Dr Muzaffar, Dr Ashraf, and Dr Akib). We thank all of them for their ever-encouraging support and continuous guidance.

We would be failing in our duty if we do not thank all the 'behind the scene people,' our parents who stood with us in tough times and all our patients who are the source of our knowledge and consented for various photographs.

We express our appreciation and gratitude to Shri Jitendar P Vij (Group Chairman), Mr Ankit Vij (Group President), Mr Tarun Duneja (Director-Publishing), Ms Samina Khan (Executive Assistant to Director-Publishing), and Mr Rajesh Sharma (Production Coordinator) of M/s Jaypee Brothers Medical Publishers (P) Ltd, New Delhi, India.

CONTENTS

Chapter

1 Introduction

Psoriasis or psoriasis vulgaris (derived from Greek words, Psora- "Itch" and sis- "action or condition") is a chronically relapsing and remitting immune mediated disorder which affects skin, scalp, nails, joints and various other organs of the body. The disorder is a chronic, recurring condition that varies in severity from minor localized patches to the involvement of whole body. It occurs in 2–4% of the general population. Psoriasis is classified as a papulosquamous disorder. It is most commonly classified according to morphologic descriptions. The variants include plaque, pustular, guttate, flexural and erythrodermic psoriasis. Psoriasis is thought to have first been described in Ancient Rome by Cornelius Celsus. The British dermatologist Thomas Bateman described a possible link between psoriasis and arthritic symptoms in 1813.[1]

The characteristic lesions of psoriasis are characterized by well-demarcated erythematous indurated scaly plaques especially over the extensor surfaces of the body. The disease is extremely variable in extent of involvement, duration, periodicity of flares, systemic involvement and response to treatment. It is widely believed that both genetic and environmental factors have a critical role in the causation of this disease.[2]

It is more common in whites and those who live farther from the equator and it is equally common in men and women. Psoriasis is more common with certain human leukocyte antigen (HLA) subtypes, but these cannot be distinguished histologically or clinically and there is no apparent difference in the response to therapy. Psoriasis can generally be divided into 2 types: Type 1 psoriasis which is characterized by a strong family history, an association with HLA-CW6 and usually presents before 40 years of age. Type 2 is not familial in presentation, has no association with HLA-CW6 and usually presents after 40 years of age.[3]

Nowadays, psoriasis vulgaris is recognised as the most prevalent autoimmune disease caused by inappropriate activation of the cellular immune system. Psoriasis affects people of all ages, but there is a strong tendency for disease onset in early life in patients with family history (i.e. who develop psoriasis due to genetic transmission). There has been a major international effort to characterise psoriasis susceptibility genes, but till date, various linkage analysis studies have failed to advance the understanding of disease pathophysiology. Unlike other common tissue-specific autoimmune diseases, psoriasis vulgaris does not have a generally accepted animal model and thus our understanding of pathogenesis of psoriasis is derived mainly from clinical studies and translational science done in patients with this disease.[4]

Points to Remember

- Psoriasis vulgaris is recognised as the most prevalent autoimmune disease caused by inappropriate activation of the cellular immune system
- It is more common in whites and those who live farther from the equator and it is equally common in men and women
- Psoriasis is classified as a papulosquamous disorder. It occurs in 2–4% of the general population
- Psoriasis is more common with certain human leukocyte antigen (HLA) subtypes, e.g. HLA-CW6
- Identification of susceptibility genes has pointed to a major role for both the innate and the adaptive immune system

REFERENCES

1. Griffiths CEM, Barker JNWN. Psoriasis, in Rook's textbook of Dermatology (8th edition), Vol 1. Wiley-Blackwell; pp. 1-60.
2. Beheet PE. Psoriasis, a brief historical review. Arch Dermatol Syphilol. 1936;33:327-34.
3. Farber EM, McClintock RP Jr. A current review of psoriasis. Calif Med. 1986;108:440-57.
4. Baker H. Psoriasis: A review. Dermatologica. 1957;150:16-25.

Chapter

2

Epidemiological Aspects of Psoriasis

The word 'prevalence' of psoriasis usually means the estimated population of people who are managing psoriasis at any given point of time (i.e. people with psoriasis). The term 'incidence' of psoriasis means the annual diagnosis rate, or the number of new cases of psoriasis diagnosed each year (i.e. getting psoriasis). Hence, these two statistical types can differ: a short disease like flu can have high annual incidence but low prevalence, but a life-long disease like diabetes has a low annual incidence but high prevalence.[1]

Psoriasis is an immune-mediated chronic disorder of the skin characterized by erythematous, indurated and scaly itchy plaques. It affects people of both sexes and of all ages and races/ethnicities. The global prevalence of psoriasis varies geographically, with the disease being more prevalent in the colder areas of the north and less prevalent in the tropics and warmer regions of the world. In European countries, psoriasis is more prevalent in residents of the colder central regions and less prevalent in residents of the southern regions. In some Asian countries, such as India, the prevalence of psoriasis is highest in the northern parts of the country. In contrast to India, China shows no difference in prevalence between the northern and southern regions. In addition to the north-to-south prevalence gradient observed within most countries, the prevalence of psoriasis also varies among different countries. Globally, the prevalence of psoriasis varies from as low as 0.03% in Japan to as high as 3.15% in USA. Differences in the reported prevalence between countries may be attributable to variations in environmental factors, genetic factors and differences in the case definition used to diagnose psoriasis in epidemiology studies.[2,3]

The incidence and prevalence of psoriasis varies according to age, gender, region and ethnicity; a combination of environmental and genetic factors is thought to be responsible for these differences. It can occur at any age, although it most commonly appears for the first time between the ages of 15 and 25 years. Psoriasis affects children also. Approximately one third of psoriasis patients report being diagnosed before the age of 20. Psoriasis affects both sexes equally.

Psoriasis is more common in countries farther from the equator, in people with inflammatory bowel disease such as Crohn's disease or ulcerative colitis, occurs most often in persons of white European ancestry and is estimated to affect 2–4% of the population of the western world. It is relatively uncommon in African Americans and is very rare or nonexistent in Inuits, Latin American Indians or Samoans.[4]

Psoriasis has a bimodal distribution of age of onset as shown by German and UK studies. The early or larger peak between 16–22 years and the later one at 57–60 years. Those individuals with an early onset disease have a severe disease and familial association. However, there is a considerable variation in the age of onset of the disease. A UK study has reported the onset of disease in 75% before the age of 46 years. The disease affects males and females equally and is morphologically similar in both the sexes.[5]

The molecular genetic basis of psoriasis is complex with evidence that multiple genes are involved. Classic genome wide linkage analysis has identified at least nine psoriasis susceptibility regions (PSORS1-9) in various chromosomes. Various association studies have shown that the most important genetic locus is PSORS1 (on chromosome 6p), which is estimated to account for up to 50% of psoriasis risk. An association between psoriasis and other loci has also been reported on chromosomes 1p (PSORS7), 1q (PSORS4), 3q (PSORS5), 4q (PSORS3), 17q (PSORS2) and 19p (PSORS6). The strength of associations between such genes and susceptibility to psoriasis, apart from PSORS1, is variable as replication of these findings has been incomplete. The difficulty of confirming psoriasis susceptibility loci may relate, in part, to heterogenity among different populations. Whereas the existence of a genetic component in psoriasis is certain, the exact location of the genes involved remains to be definitely determined.[6]

For many years it was thought that psoriasis was purely a skin disorder, but more recent studies have shown that immunosuppressive agents reduce psoriasis. The current model is that psoriasis is a complex autoimmune disease in which T cells are mistakenly activated, triggering other immune responses. Various environmental triggers such as trauma, stress, infection, climate changes, and drugs, including beta-blockers and lithium activate the disease in genetically predisposed individuals. The genetic basis of the disease is well established. Studies have shown that 30% of psoriasis patients have a first-degree relative with the condition. In cases where both a parent and one child are affected, siblings have a 50% chance of developing psoriasis.[7]

Points to Remember

- Psoriasis has a bimodal distribution of age of onset, the early or larger peak between 16–22 years and the later one at 57–60 years. The most common sites of involvement are the scalp, elbows and knees, followed by the nails, hands, feet and trunk
- Studies have shown that 30% of psoriasis patients have a first-degree relative with the condition
- Psoriasis is a complex autoimmune disease in which T cells are mistakenly activated, triggering other immune responses

REFERENCES

1. Lomholt G. Prevalence of skin disease in a population: A census study from the Faroe islands. Dan Med Bull. 1964;11:1-7.
2. Smith AE, Kassab JY, Rowland Payne CM, Beer WE. Bimodality in age of onset of psoriasis, in both patients and their relatives. Dermatology. 1993;186:181-6.
3. Ambady BM, Gopinath T, Nair BHK. Psoriasis. Indian J Dermatol Venereol Leprol. 1961;23:27-34.
5. Henseler T, Christophers E. Psoriasis of early and late onset: Characterization of two types of psoriasis vulgaris. J Am Acad Dermatol. 1985;13:450-6.
5. Farber EM, Nall ML. Epidemiology, natural history and genetics. In: Roenigk HH, Maibach HI, editors. Psoriasis. New York: Marcel Dekker; 1998.pp.107-58.
6. Watson W, Cann HM, Farber EM, et al. The genetics of psoriasis. Arch Dermatol. 1972;105:197-207.
7. Krueger G, Ellis CN. Psoriasis-recent advances in understanding its pathogenesis and treatment. J Am Acad Dermatol. 2005;53:94-100.

Chapter

3

Psoriasis in India

Psoriasis is a chronic or chronically relapsing and remitting disease of the skin characterized by hyperproliferation and inflammation of the epidermal and dermal components of the skin. The typical clinical picture is of well-defined, erythematous, indurated and itchy scaly plaques located predominantly on the extensor surfaces and scalp consistent with the clinical variant known as psoriasis vulgaris. Several different morphological forms are also known to be manifested in the skin. In addition to the skin, the disease affects nails, joints and also rarely the mucosal surfaces. Psoriasis is known to affect 1–2% of the world population. The disease is known for its wide geographical variations due to genetic, racial, geographical and environmental reasons. The prevalence in United States of America is as high as 4.6–4.7%. A negligible prevalence in West Africans, Japanese, North American Indians and Eskimos is seen (attributable to the high content of essential fatty acids in the diet of the latter perhaps).[1] Prevalence studies from India are mostly hospital-based. Okhandiar et al. in a hospital-based study collected a comprehensive data from various medical colleges located in Dibrugarh, Calcutta, Patna, Darbhanga, Lucknow, New Delhi and Amritsar. They found that the incidence of psoriasis among total skin patients ranged between 0.44 and 2.2%, with an overall incidence of 1.02%. They noted that the incidence in Amritsar (2.2%) was higher as compared to other centers in Eastern India and speculated that it may be related to different environmental conditions (extremes of temperature), dietary habits and genetic differences. Male to female ratio (2.46:1) was very high which could not be clearly accounted for. Highest incidence was noted in the age group of 20–39 years and the mean age of onset in males and females was comparable.[2] In a study conducted by Masood Q and Hassan I in Srinagar, the prevalence of psoriasis in patients attending the dermatology out patient department of SMHS Hospital; the main tertiary care hospital of Kashmir valley, was reported to be 3.4%.[3]

In a study from a tertiary health care center from North India, psoriasis patients accounted for 2.3% of the total dermatology outpatients. Of the total psoriasis patients, 67% were men and 33% were women, male to female ratio being 2.03:1. Ages of patients ranged from infancy to eighth decade, mean age being 33.6 years. Children accounted for 4.4% of total psoriasis patients. Women had slightly lower mean age of onset (27.6 years) compared to men (30.9 years).[2]

In yet another study from North India, Bedi TR reported the prevalence of psoriasis to be 0.8% among the skin patients but the sample size of the study was very small. Male to female sex ratio was 2.5:1. In this study, it was observed that females had lower mean age of onset compared to males. In a subsequent study by Bedi TR which included larger number (530) of subjects, the prevalence of psoriasis among dermatology outpatients was found to be 2.8%, whereas the male to female ratio continued to be the same.[4,5]

So, it can be concluded from various studies that in India the prevalence of psoriasis varies from 0.44% to 2.8%, it is twice more common in males compared to females and most of the patients are in their third or fourth decade at the time of presentation. These studies are limited by the absence of commonly accepted and validated diagnostic criteria. Furthermore, there is basically no reliable information on the time trends of the disease.

Points to Remember

- In India, the prevalence of psoriasis varies from 0.44 to 2.8%, it is twice more common in males compared to females and most of the patients are in their third or fourth decade at the time of presentation
- Children account for 4–5% of total psoriasis patients in India

REFERENCES

1. Sharma T, Sepha GC. Psoriasis-clinical study. Indian J Dermatol Venereol Leprol. 1964;30:191-7.
2. Dogra S, Yadav S. Psoriasis in India: Prevalance and pattern. Indian J Dermatol Venereol Leprol. 2010;76: 595-601.
3. Masood Q, Hassan I. Pattern of skin disorders in Kashmir valley. Indian J Dermatol. 2002;47(3):147-8.
4. Bedi TR. Psoriasis in North India-geographical variations. Dermatologica. 1977;155:310-4.
5. Bedi TR. Psoriasis in Children. Indian J Dermatol Venereol Leprol. 1979;45:410-3.

Chapter

4

Genetic and Familial Factors in Psoriasis

The role of genetic factors in psoriasis has been provided by various genome-wide association studies,and is now well recognised. Various genetic studies have shown that psoriasis is more common in the first and second degree relatives of psoriasis patients than in the general population. It has been estimated that an approximately 30% of patients with psoriasis vulgaris have an affected first degree relative. The risk is higher in monozygotic twins, as shown by various concordance studies. Psoriasis vulgaris is known to be associated with certain HLA antigens (HLA-Cw6 allele mostly) and complement factors but most of the studies published are in western populations with only little information about Indians. Chablani et al. in a study of 67 psoriasis subjects from Western India found an association with HLA A1, B17 and Cw6, but not with B13 antigens. Pitchappan et al. reported association of HLA Bw57 and DR7 with psoriasis vulgaris in South India. Rani et al. showed that Cw FNx010602 was the main allele that had high frequency in psoriasis patients in North India.[1,2]

HLA-Cw6 is strongly linked with the age of onset of psoriasis. In one series, HLA-cw6 was expressed in 90% of psoriasis patients with early-onset psoriasis, in 50% of those with late-onset psoriasis and only in 7% of a control population.

Psoriatic arthritis is now believed to be a distinct disorder rather than an association/ complication with psoriasis, although the two disorders share certain HLA alleles. The association of psoriasis and psoriatic arthritis (PsA) with alleles in the MHC region has been recognised for over three decades and currently there are a number of association studies for both these disorders with HLA alleles. For instance class I antigens HLA-B13, HLA-B17 and its split HLA-B57 and HLA-Cw6 have consistently shown a positive association with psoriasis across various population studies. The presence of HLA Cw 0602 is associated with more severe and early-onset psoriasis and is found in 100% of patients with guttate psoriasis. Meanwhile, HLA-Cw*0602 is increased among those with psoriatic arthritis (PsA) and is also associated with an earlier age of onset of psoriasis. HLA-B27, HLA-B38 and HLA-B39 have also consistently been noted to have an increased frequency in psoriatic arthritis (PsA) cases compared with controls. With respect to disease expression, HLA-B27 is associated with back involvement, while HLA-B38 and HLA-B39 occurs more frequently among patients with peripheral polyarthritis.[3]

With the advent of genome-wide association studies, the genetic basis of psoriasis has become more evident. In order to elucidate the genetic determinants, the researchers have now shifted the focus, at regions outside the MHC region. Single nucleotide polymorphism technology and genotyping, have greatly contributed to the genetic pathogenesis of psoriasis.[4]

Genetic predisposition has a significant role in the etiopathogenesis of psoriasis as familial clustering of the cases has been observed. Familial incidence is greater in childhood psoriasis compared to adult-onset psoriasis follow-up. Farber and Nall reported familial occurrence in 36% of their patients, with a high concordance rate among monozygotic twins. A two- to three-fold increased risk of psoriasis was noted in monozygotic twins compared to the dizygotic twins,implying that genetic factors are important. The distribution of lesions, severity and the age of onset were similar in the monozygotic twins compared to the dizygotic twins in whom these features differed.[5]

Indian studies report lower familial incidence of the disease. Bedi reported positive family history of psoriasis in 14% of their patients whereas Kaur et al. reported family history in only 2% of their patients. First-degree relatives were affected in 84% of the cases whereas second-degree relatives were affected in 12% of cases. There are only few studies which have made a record of family history of psoriasis in their patients, so definite statistical data on familial incidence is not available.[6]

Thus, there is a clear genetic contribution to psoriasis and psoriatic arthritis (PsA). Although there are distinct genetic differences between these two disorders, but epidemiological and immunological evidence suggests that some genetic determinants are likely to be shared between these two diseases. With the strong genetic contribution to psoriasis and psoriatic arthritis (PsA), coupled with rapidly advancing linkage and association studies, elucidation of the major genetic determinants of these diseases will be possible in near future.[7]

Points to Remember

- Genetic predisposition has a significant role in the etiopathogenesis of psoriasis and familial clustering of the cases has been observed
- There is a clear genetic contribution to psoriasis and psoriatic arthritis (PsA). Indian studies report lower familial incidence of the disease
- The presence of HLA-Cw*0602 is associated with more severe and early-onset psoriasis and has been found in approximately 100% of patients with guttate psoriasis
- Psoriasis is a chronic, immune-mediated disorder that results from a polygenic predisposition combined with environmental triggers, e.g. trauma, infections and medication.

REFERENCES

1. Elder JT, Nair RP, Guo SW, Henseler T, Christophers E, Voorhees JJ. The genetics of psoriasis. Arch Dermatol. 1994;130:216-24.
2. Ameen M, Barker JN. Genetics. Psoriasis. In: Gordon KB, Ruderman EM, editors. Psoriasis and Psoriatic arthritis, 1st edn. New York: Springer; 2005.pp.3-12.
3. Bowcock AM, Cookson WO. The genetics of psoriasis, psoriatic arthritis and atopic dermatitis. Hum Mol Genet. 2004;13:R43-55.
4. Christophers E, Henseler T. Psoriasis type I and type II as subtypes of nonpustular psoriasis. In: Roenigk H, Maibach H, eds. Psoriasis. New York: Marcel Dekker; 1990.pp.15-21.
5. Elder JT, Nair RP, Henseler T, Jenisch S, Stuart P, Chia N, et al. The genetics of psoriasis 2001: the odyssey continues. Arch Dermatol. 2001;137:1447-54.
6. Kaur I, Kumar B, Sharma VK. Epidemiology of psoriasis in a clinic from North India. Indian J Dermatol Venereol Leprol. 1986;52:208-12.
7. Kreuger JG, Bowcock A. Psoriasis pathophysiology: current concepts of pathogenesis. Ann Rheum Dis. 2005;64(suppl II):ii30-6.

Chapter

5 Etiology and Pathogenesis

Psoriasis is an immune mediated skin disorder with multifactorial and a complex etiology. Psoriasis is considered to be a disease with prominent involvement of T cells, keratinocytes and various secreted cytokines. Various factors which have been suggested to play a key role in the pathogenesis are T cells, antigen presenting cells (APC's), keratinocytes, Langerhans' cells, macrophages, natural killer (NK) cells, an array of Th1 type cytokines, certain growth factors like vascular endothelial growth factor (VEGF), keratinocyte growth factor (KGF) and others. It has been hypothesized that the disease starts with the activation of T cell by an unknown antigen, which leads to secretion of an array of cytokines by activated T cells, inflammatory cells, and keratinocytes. This leads to activation of langerhan's cells, which migrate from skin to lymph nodes presenting the antigen to nodal nai've T cells (cells that have not been activated by antigen previously). The T cells activated by nonantigen-dependent mechanism may, however become antigen-specific memory cells that react with a cross-reactive autoantigen, such as keratin (molecular mimicry). The characteristic lesion of psoriasis (well-defined erythematous, indurated, scaly plaque) is due to the hyperproliferation of the keratinocyte. The genetic background of the disease may be suggested from the fact that a positive family history has been reported by 35–90% of patients with psoriasis, concordance rate is 63–73% in monozygotic twins, as compared to 17–20% in dizygotic twins. Classic genome-wide linkage analysis has identified at least nine psoriasis susceptibility regions (PSORS1-9) in different chromosomal locations.[1,2]

With recent advances in molecular biology, psoriasis is regarded as a T-cell driven disease. But the fundamental question which remains is: Whether psoriasis represents a fundamental disease of skin, or the immune system? The role of T cells, antigen-presenting cells, keratinocytes, Langerhans' cell, macrophages, natural killer cells, an array of Th1 type cytokines, certain growth factors like VEGF, KGF and others have been suggested to play a key role in pathogenesis of psoriasis. Currently a wide array of treatment modalities are available for psoriasis, but with every treatment there is a possibility of remission only.[3] There is a need to review our current concept and understanding of the pathogenesis of psoriasis. Lack of a clear pathogenetic mechanism especially in remissions, makes it very difficult to manage the disease on long-term basis. In the past decade researchers have come up with new factors that may be involved in the pathogenesis of disease, but they have failed to establish a pathogenetic model that incorporates all the factors, due to the lack of an animal model.[4]

1. *Role of T-cells and dendritic cells in the pathogenesis:* Several cell types have been implicated in the pathogenesis and maintenance of psoriatic lesions. The association of psoriasis with particular MHC alleles, such as HLA-Cw6, as well as the presence of specific T-cell subsets within the epidermis and dermis of lesional skin is well documented. Most of the epidermal

T-cells are CD8+, whereas the dermal infiltrate is a mixture of CD4+ and CD8+ cells. T-cell activation has been suggested to play a key role in the pathogenesis of psoriasis. It is widely believed that abnormal regulation of T cells coupled with interaction between keratinocytes and a complex cytokine network is involved in the pathogenesis of this intriguing disease. Few studies have suggested that the primary defect resides in keratinocytes, thus it is believed that any physical or chemical injury to the defective keratinocytes could activate synthesis and release of cytokines thereby resulting in antigen-independent activation of T lymphocytes. This would further lead to release of additional cytokines followed by proliferation of keratinocytes, T lymphocytes and inflammation. Chang et al. have demonstrated that cytokines secreted by psoriatic epidermal cells potentiate T lymphocyte activation to a greater extent than cytokines secreted from normal epidermal cells. It is also postulated that only psoriatic keratinocytes respond to activated T cell signals with hyperproliferation, because of their specific receptors or signal-transducing mechanisms. Further normal keratinocytes do not respond to psoriatic T cell supernatants.[5]

Dendritic cells have been demonstrated in lesional psoriatic skin and because of their potent immunostimulatory capacity, they are believed to be involved in the pathogenesis of psoriasis. There is an increased number of dermal dendritic cells in psoriatic skin and they have an enhanced ability to activate T cells. These cells have an ability to differentiate into potent proinflammatory dendritic cells that produce inducible nitric oxide synthase (iNOS) and TNF-α. The role of dendritic cells in psoriasis has been validated by the presence of a prominent genomic dendritic cell signature and the decrease of dendritic cells during effective targeted therapy.[6]

According to some studies, the basement membrane (BM) structures are altered and a complex network of cytokines, mainly Th1 type, are involved in various stages of pathogenesis. The role of T-cells has also been established due to the beneficial effect of drugs/agents which affect T-cell function. Alefacept (a biological agent) which binds to CD2 on T cells, blocks the LFA-3/CD2 interaction. Alefacept also binds to FcgRIII IgG receptors on NK cells and macrophages, resulting in apoptosis of those T cells expressing high levels of CD2. Efalizumab, a biological agent is an antibody directed against the alpha subunit of LFA-1. Etanercept and infliximab (biological agents) which are competitive inhibitors of tumor necrosis factor-alpha (TNF-α), are the latest treatment modalities for psoriasis.[7]

2. *Role of keratinocytes in the pathogenesis:* Psoriasis is believed to be a multifactorial disease where both genetic and environmental factors act together. Psoriasis is characterized by hyperproliferation and abnormal differentiation of epidermal keratinocytes, T lymphocyte infiltration and various changes in the dermis, such as, angiogenesis, dilatation and high endothelial venule formation. The cell cycle time of hyperproliferating psoriatic keratinocytes is short. While maturation and shedding of keratinocytes takes 28 days in normal epidermis, it occurs in 4 days in psoriatic epidermis. Growth factors, released by various cell types, are believed to stimulate the increased proliferation of keratinocytes. The role of keratinocytes in the pathogenesis of psoriasis is also suggested by the fact that various drugs which act on keratinocytes help in the amelioration of psoriasis; example being vitamin D3 analogues and retinoids. Calcipotriol, a vitamin D3 analog and retinoids, the natural and synthetic vitamin A derivatives, modulate keratinocyte hyperproliferation and differentiation. Cyclosporine, an immunomodulator and immunosuppressive agent

has strong antiproliferative effects on human epidermal keratinocytes in addition to its suppressive effects on T cells.[8]

3. *Role of blood vessels and angiogenesis in the pathogenesis of psoriasis:*[9] Prominent angiogenesis is observed in the plaques of psoriasis. There is increased expression of VEGF, and anti-VEGF therapy leads to improvement in psoriasis in experimental mouse models of psoriasis. Keratinocytes are thought to be a major source of pro-angiogenic cytokines (VEGF, IL-8) but the precise mechanism for angiogenesis in psoriasis is still unknown. In a developing psoriatic plaque, endothelial cells swell and become activated showing prominent Golgi apparatus and Weibel–Palade bodies. Activated endothelial cells migrate, sprout and lay down a basement membrane with pericytes for structural support to form novel vessel networks. Activation and swelling of endothelial cells results in widening of the intercellular spaces and dermal blood vessels dilate. The lesional capillary loops adopt a venous phenotype, including bridged fenestrations and express E-selectin, making it easier for leukocytes to migrate into the skin. Although angiogenesis may not be the primary event in the pathogenesis of psoriasis, understanding the pathways leading to angiogenesis may help in finding novel antipsoriatic drugs. In fact, vitamin D analogues, retinoids and cyclosporine all possess anti-angiogenic activity as well as antiproliferative and anti-inflammatory effects.
   Despite the clear familial aggregation of psoriasis, the precise inheritance model has been elusive till date. Despite the advances made in the field of molecular biology, currently most researchers have come to the conclusion that psoriasis belongs to the group of complex diseases, the inheritance being multifactorial—genetic variants in multiple genes interact both with each other as well as with the environment. Several disease susceptibility loci (PSORS1-9) have been suggested as predisposing factors.
4. *Role of cytokine mediators in the pathogenesis of psoriasis:*[10,11] Cytokines are low molecular weight glycoproteins or small polypeptides that act as signaling molecules to orchestrate host inflammation, defense, tissue repair and remodeling, growth, fibrosis, angiogenesis and control of neoplasm. Although a complex and multi-dimensional network of several cytokines has been found to be involved in pathophysiology of psoriasis, none of these alone can be considered to be the causative. There is a predominance of Th1-type cytokines (IFN-γ, IL-2 and TNF-α) in the psoriatic plaques. Recently another chemokine CX3CL1 called fractalkine (in humans) or neurotactin (in mice) has been identified in psoriasis. CX3CL1 is produced as a long protein (with 373-amino acids in humans) with an extended mucin-like stalk and a chemokine domain on top. The mucin-like stalk permits it to bind to the surface of certain cells. However, a soluble (90 kD) version of this chemokine has also been observed. Soluble CX3CL1 chemokine attracts T cells and monocytes, while the cell-bound chemokine promotes strong adhesion of leukocytes to activated endothelial cells, where it is primarily expressed. Fractalkine binding to its seven-transmembrane domain G protein coupled receptor CX3CR1 triggers signalling, but it also directly mediates cell adhesion.
   Chemokines are important mediators in the trafficking of leukocytes and the increased presence of several chemokines in psoriatic lesions has been well documented. CXCL8 is thought to mediate the infiltration of neutrophils into psoriatic lesions. CCL17, CCL20, CCL27 and CXCL9-11 are implicated in attracting T cells into the psoriatic lesions. A pDC-attracting chemokine, chemerin, is increased in psoriatic skin and might contribute to the early recruitment of pDCs into psoriatic lesions.

There is no question that advances in understanding the cellular immunology and biology of psoriasis, when coupled with the biotechnology revolution and rapid advances derived from human genetic studies of autoimmunity, have enhanced insights into the causation and treatment of psoriasis. The disease starts with the activation of T lymphocytes with an unknown antigen or gene product. T cell activation depends on its binding with APC (antigen presenting cell). T cells express the cell receptor known as TCR (T cell receptor), which recognizes the peptide being presented by the APC in the grove of MHC complex. The antigen stimulated activation leads to the conversion of nai've T-cells into an antigen specific cell, which may develop into a memory cell that circulate in the body. After the activation of T cells, a cascade of cytokines viz. GM-CSF (granulocyte macrophage colony stimulating factor), EGF, IL-1, IL-6, IL-8, IL-12, IL-17, IL-23, Fractalkine, TNF-α, etc. are secreted by the activated T Cells. Due to effect of these cytokines there is keratinocyte proliferation, neutrophil migration, potentiation of Th-1 type response, angiogenesis, up-regulation of adhesion molecules and epidermal hyperplasia. Currently newer therapies are in pipeline, including an anti-IL23/22 fully humanized antibody,which has shown promise in treating psoriasis, but results of clinical trials will only prove its efficacy as long-term cure.

Points to Remember

- Psoriasis is a multifactorial skin disease with a complex pathogenesis
- Hyperproliferation of keratinocytes, T-cell activation, angiogenesis and cytokine mediators are believed to be involved in the pathogenesis of psoriasis
- Whether psoriasis represents a fundamental disease of skin, or the immune system has been debated for several years

REFERENCES

1. Das RP, Jain AK, Ramesh V. Current concepts in the pathogenesis of psoriasis. Indian J Dermatol. 2009;54:7-12.
2. Henseler T. Genetics of psoriasis. Arch Dermatol Res. 1998;290:463-76.
3. Elder JT, Nair RP, Henseler T, Jenisch S, Stuart P, Chia N, et al . The genetics of psoriasis 2001: The odyssey continues. Arch Dermatol. 2001;137:1447-54.
4. Krueger JG, Bowcock A. Psoriasis pathophysiology: Current concepts of pathogenesis. Ann Rheum Dis. 2005;64:ii30-6.
5. Mehlis SL, Gordon KB. The immunology of psoriasis and biologic immunotherapy. J Am Acad Dermatol. 2003;49:44-50.
6. Chamlan F, Lowes MA, Lin SL. Alefacept reduces infiltrating T cells, activated dendritic cells, and inflammatory genes in psoriasis vulgaris. Proc Natl Acad Sci USA. 2005;102:2075-80.
7. Bos JD, De Rie MA. The pathogenesis of psoriasis: Immunological facts and speculations. Immunol Today. 1999;20:40-6.
8. Voorhees JJ. Pathophysiology of psoriasis. Annu Rev Med. 1977;28:467-73.
9. Sugiyama H, Gyulai R, Toichi E. Dysfunctional blood and target tissue CD4+ CD25 high regulatory T cells in psoriasis mechanism underlying unrestrained pathogenic effector T-cell proliferation. J Immunol. 2005;174:164-73.
10. Raychaudhuri SP, Jiang WY, Farber EM. Cellular localization of fractalkine at sites of inflammation:antigen presenting cells in psoriasis express high levels of fractalkine. Br J Dermatol. 2001;144:1105-13.
11. Rottman JB, Smith TL, Ganley KG. Potential role of the chemokine receptors CXCR3, CXCR4 and the integrin αEβ7 in the pathogenesis of psoriasis vulgaris. Lab invest. 2001;81:335-47.

Chapter

6 Histology and Pathology

Psoriasis is especially a clinical diagnosis, but histopathology becomes essential in cases of diagnostic uncertainty and unusual presentations of psoriasis. The histologic features commonly present in psoriasis include acanthosis, uniform elongation of the rete ridges, parakeratosis and orthokeratosis, loss of the granular cell layer and the formation of spongiform pustules and parakeratotic microabscesses.

In the epidermis, the rete ridges are narrow towards the surface and broad at the base. Bridges may form among some of these ridges. The papillary dermis is broadened and clubbed near the surface. The capillary vessels within the superficial dermis are slightly dilated and may have associated chronic inflammation. Neutrophils extravasate from these capillaries and are found in the thinned superficial epidermis (spongiform pustules of Kogoj, seen in stratum spinosum). These neutrophils eventually aggregate in the parakeratotic layer, forming the Munro microabscess (in stratum corneum), which is characteristic of this condition.

Mitotic activity, commonly seen only in the basal cells, is typically increased in psoriasis. Mitotic figures are present in the parabasal (prickle cell) layers (Figs 6.1 and 6.2).

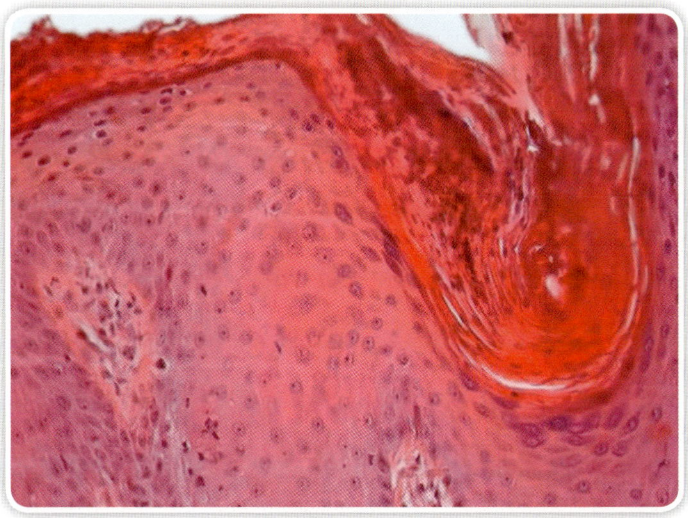

FIG. 6.1: High power view of a psoriatic plaque showing hyperkeratosis and acanthosis
(*Courtesy:* Dr Syed Imtiyaz, MD, Pathology, GMC Srinagar)

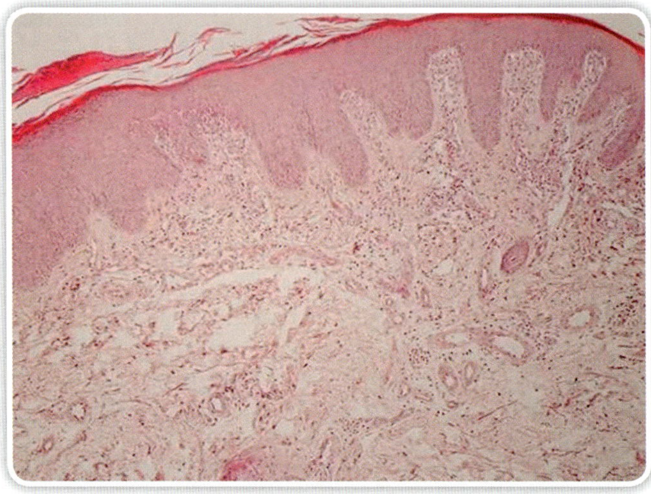

FIG. 6.2: Low-power view of a psoriatic plaque
(*Courtesy:* Dr Syed Imtiyaz, MD, Pathology, GMC Srinagar)

Changes in fully developed psoriatic plaques: There is hyperkeratosis, parakeratosis, focal orthokeratosis and munro microabscess formation, absent or greatly thinned granular layer, spongiform pustules in the Malphigian layer, hyperplasia with elongation of the rete ridges and suprapapillary epidermal thinning. The rete ridges are narrow at the top and often clubbed, branched or fused at their bases, with mononuclear leukocytic infiltrate in the lower half of epidermis. Dilated tortuous papillary blood vessels almost touch the undersurface of thinnend suprapapillary epidermis and are surrounded by a mixed mononuclear and neutrophilic infiltrate, as well as extravasated erythrocytes. Invasion of the epidermis with leukocytes is seen particularly in the suprapapillary epidermis (Fig. 6.3).[1,2]

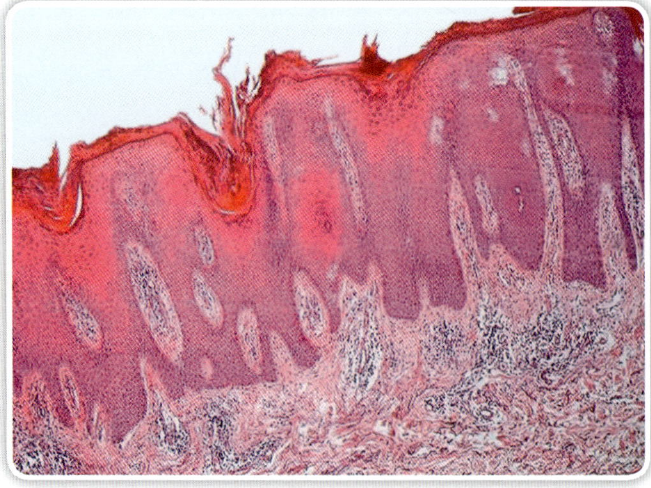

FIG. 6.3: Histopathological picture of a fully developed psoriatic plaque
(*Courtesy:* Dr Syed Imtiyaz, MD, Pathology, GMC Srinagar)

REFERENCES

1. Lever WF, Schaumburg-Lever G. Histopathology of the Skin (Seventh edition). Philadelphia: JB Lippincott; 1990.pp.156-61.
2. Bacharach-Buhles M, Gammals EL, Panz B. In psoriasis the epidermis including the subepidermal vascular plexus grows downwards into the dermis. Br J Dermatol. 1997;136:97-101.

Chapter 7

Clinical Presentations of Psoriasis

There are varied clinical presentations of psoriasis. Broadly, it has been classified into nonpustular and pustular psoriasis. There are further clinical phenotypes of each. It is important to recognize precisely the clinical subtype as it has implications on the choice of treatment modality and also reflects upon the disease activity. Most common clinical type is the classic chronic plaque type psoriasis (psoriasis vulgaris). But even same clinical subtype can behave differently in different individuals.

Henseler and Christopher on the basis of phenotype database of 2147 patients, recognized two distinct patient cohorts. One cohort had early onset (type I) of psoriasis in the second decade and the other cohort had late onset (type II) of the disease in the fifth decade. Early-onset cohort had more widespread and recurrent disease and also higher number had affected parents compared to late-onset cohort.

There are only few studies from India which have analyzed the clinical spectrum of the disease in psoriasis patients. Okhandiar et al. collected epidemiological data of 116 psoriasis patients from various medical colleges. They found that the extensors (93%) were the most common site of involvement followed by the scalp (88%). Face, palms, soles and nails were affected in one third of the cases. Inverse psoriasis was uncommon. None of their patient had mucosal involvement and also they did not comment on the morphological types of psoriasis in their patients.[1,2]

Bedi in an Indian study analyzed data of 530 psoriasis patients seen over a period of five years. Chronic plaque type psoriasis was the most common (90%) clinical phenotype. The most common sites of involvement in descending order of frequency were trunk, limbs, scalp, face, palms, soles and flexures. The second most common clinical phenotype was palmoplantar psoriasis followed by flexural psoriasis. The guttate psoriasis, mucosal involvement and psoriatic erythroderma was noticed to be uncommon.[3]

Kaur et al. in an another study reported scalp (25%) as the most common first site of involvement followed by legs (20.6%) and arms (11.7%). Oral (0.7%) and genital (0.4%) mucosal involvement was found to be uncommon. Chronic plaque type psoriasis (93%) was the most common clinical phenotype. Palmoplantar pustulosis, guttate and erythrodermic variants accounted for less than 2% of cases each. Generalized pustular, isolated nail, flexural and arthropathic forms were very uncommon.

The pattern of postinflammatory pigmentation following clearance of lesions was reported by Kaur et al. They noted that psoriatic lesions cleared leaving no dyspigmentation in majority of the cases, while hyperpigmentation and hypopigmentation followed clearance of lesions in 9.7% and 7.3% of the patients, respectively.

Two studies by Kaur et al. have presented the data on severity of disease in their patients. In the initial study which included 782 patients, the extent of disease was 50% body surface area (BSA) involvement in two-third of patients, 50–70% BSA involvement in 15% and less in the rest. Recent study comprising of 1220 psoriasis patients reported, <25% BSA involvement in three-fourth patients, one fifth had 26–50% and <10% had >50% BSA involvement. There are very scarce Indian studies to provide data on the severity of disease among psoriasis patients based on PASI scores.[4]

Besides being cosmetically disabling, psoriasis leads to morbidity due to pruritus and burning sensation in many patients. Okhandiar et al. found pruritus to be present in 95% of their cases, whereas burning and smarting sensation was seen in around 15% cases. Bedi noted itching to be a significant complaint in 81% of the patients. Kaur et al. found that burning and stiffness were uncommon (1%) whereas pruritus was complained by 65% patients. So, the results of various studies suggest that psoriasis is definitely a pruriginous disorder adding to the morbidity of this dermatosis.

Relapses are common and the pattern of relapses are also varied in different individuals. Some have early and frequent relapses and others have long-term remissions of their disease process with infrequent relapses. There is scarcity of data on the relapse pattern of psoriasis from India. Kaur et al. reported that the duration of remission varied widely from two weeks to nine years in their patients but 4% of their patients never had complete remission of their disease.

Bedi noted seasonal variation in 46% patients, half of whom felt worsening in winters. Similarly, Kaur et al. reported seasonal variation in half of their patients, with 43% reporting improvement in summer and 7% in winter.[5]

Clinical signs useful in the identification of psoriatic lesions include:[6,7]

- Koebner phenomenon, which is the occurrence of new psoriatic lesions at the site of skin injury (Fig. 7.1).
- Woronoff's ring, which is a ring of peripheral blanching skin around a psoriatic plaque (believed to result due to local prostaglandins, PGE2).
- Auspitz's sign, which are small bleeding points seen upon lifting of a psoriatic scale (due to suprapapillary thinning) (Fig. 7.2).

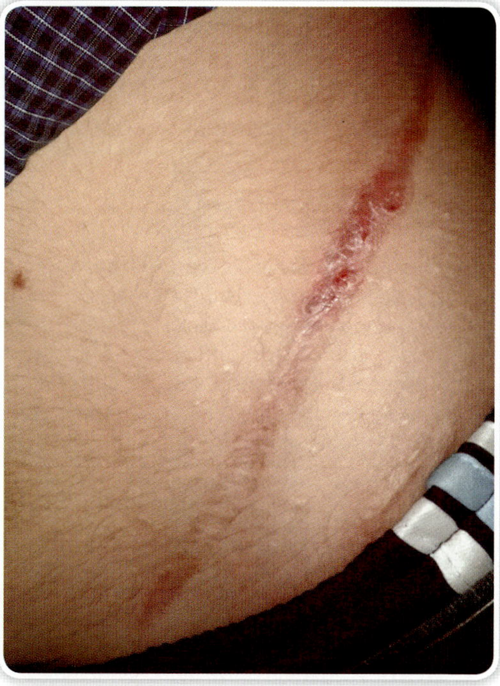

FIG. 7.1: Psoriatic plaque overlying a surgical scar (Koebner's phenomenon)

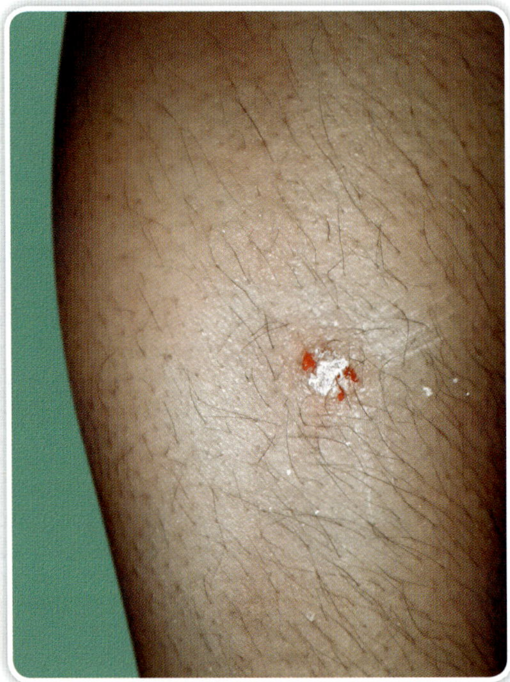

FIG. 7.2: Pin point bleeding following scraping of a psoriatic lesion (Positive auspit'z sign)

Points to Remember

- There are varied clinical presentations of psoriasis. Most common clinical type is the classic chronic plaque type psoriasis. But even same clinical subtype can behave differently in different individuals
- It is important to recognize precisely the clinical subtype as it has implications on the choice of treatment modality and also reflects upon the disease activity
- Relapses are common and the patterns of relapses are also varied in different individuals. Some have early and frequent relapses and others have long-term remissions of their disease process with infrequent relapses

REFERENCES

1. Sharma T, Sepha GC. Psoriasis-clinical study. Indian J Dermatol Venereol. 1964;30:191-7.
2. Dogra S, Yadav S. Psoriasis in India. Prevalance and pattern. Indian J Dermatol Venereol Leprol. 2010;76: 595-601.
3. Bedi TR. Psoriasis in North India-geographical variations. Dermatologica. 1977;155:310-4.
4. Kaur I, Kumar B, Sharma VK. Epidemiology of psoriasis in a clinic from North India. Indian J Dermatol Venereol Leprol. 1986;52:208-12.
5. Rosenberg EW, Noah PW. The Koebner phenomenon and the microbial basis of psoriasis. J Am Acad Dermatol. 1988;18:151-8.
6. Penneys NS, Ziboh V, Simon P, et al. Pathogenesis of Woronoff's ring in psoriasis. Arch Dermatol. 1976;112: 955-7.
7. Bernhard JD. Auspitz sign is not sensitive or specific for psoriasis. J Am Acad Dermatol. 1990;22:1079-81.

Chapter

8 Types of Psoriasis

Psoriasis has a number of clinical variants that differ in severity, location, longevity, shape, pattern, cause and treatment. Patients may experience more than one type at the same time. The different types of psoriasis are fairly distinct and are listed below.

TYPES OF PSORIASIS[1]

- Plaque psoriasis (psoriasis vulgaris)
- Flexural or inverse
- Guttate or eruptive
- Pustular
- Palmoplantar
- Erythrodermic
- Scalp
- Nail
- Acral
- Seborrhoeic
- Rupioid, elephantine and ostraceous psoriasis.

Plaque Psoriasis (Psoriasis Vulgaris)

Plaque psoriasis is the most common variant, observed in about 90% of patients. The red or salmon-coloured papulosquamous plaques are well delineated from the surrounding skin. They may be thick or thin, large or small. Classic sites of plaque involvement are the extensor aspects of elbows and knees, the scalp, shins, the lumbosacral region and the umbilicus. The involvement of face is uncommon. The plaques can develop from small papular lesions that converge to form larger plaques. In active psoriasis, the rim of the plaque expands and the center of it clears, forming a typical plaque known as annular psoriasis. With the inactive form of plaque psoriasis, lesions remain the same size even without treatment (Figs 8.1 to 8.26).

The active form has a better prognosis than the inactive form. The Koebner phenomenon describes active inflammatory psoriasis where new lesions develop at sites of trauma and pressure.[2]

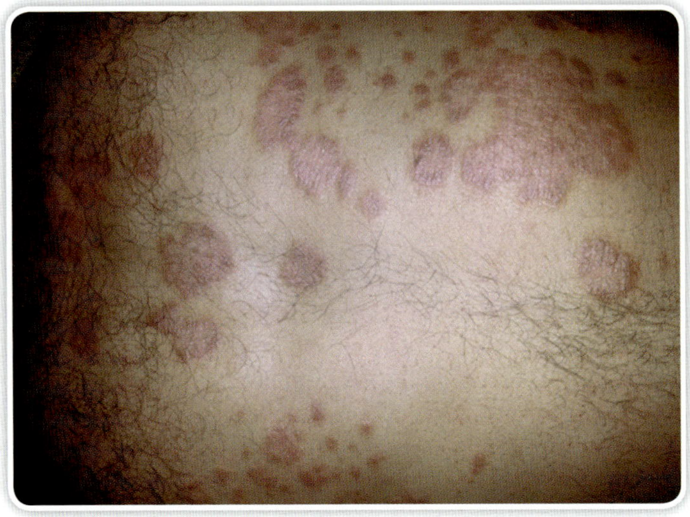

FIG. 8.1: Lesions of psoriasis vulgaris involving the trunk

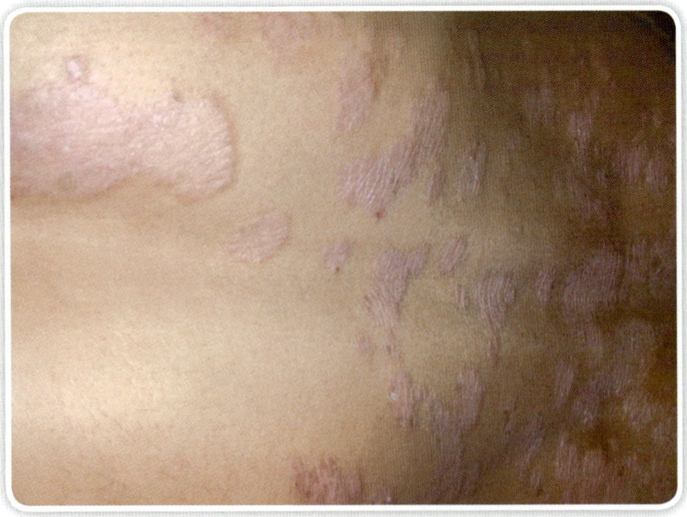

FIG. 8.2: Characteristic plaques of psoriasis involving the back in an adult

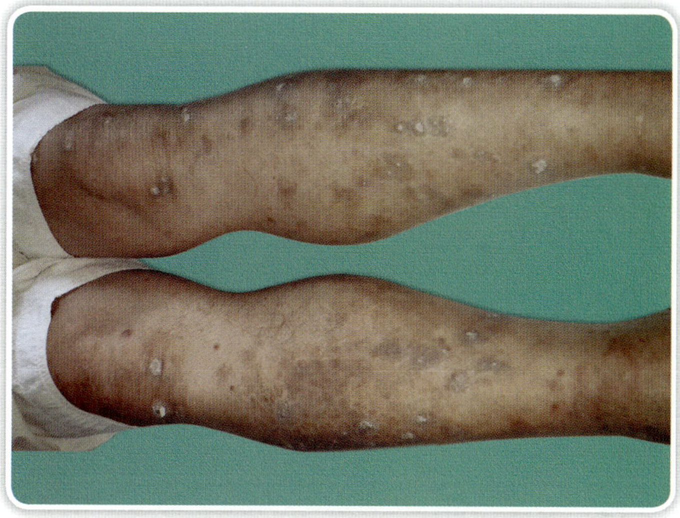

FIG. 8.3: Psoriatic plaques over both legs in a 50 year old male patient. The patient was on topical treatment

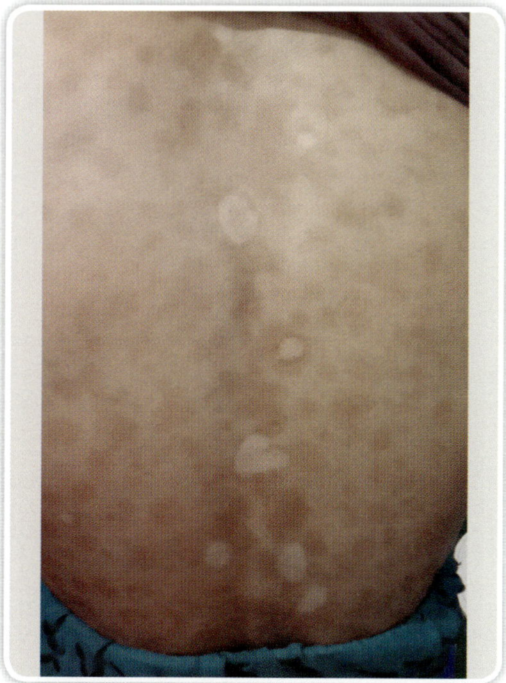

FIG. 8.4: Resolving psoriatic lesions in a patient. Note both hypo- as well as hyperpigmentation

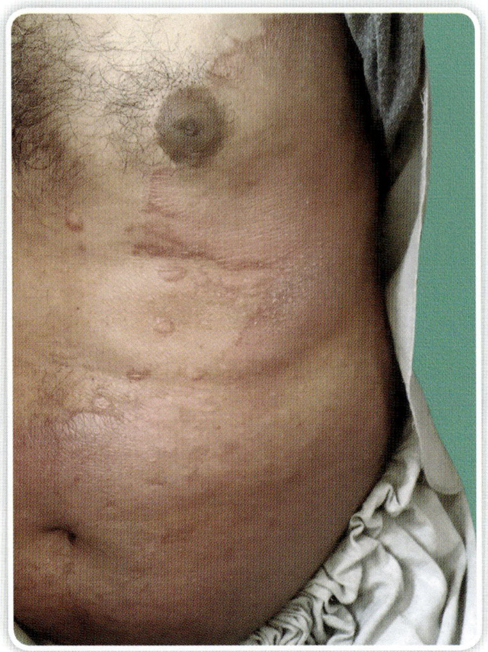

FIG. 8.5: Large irregular plaques of psoriasis over chest and abdomen in a male patient

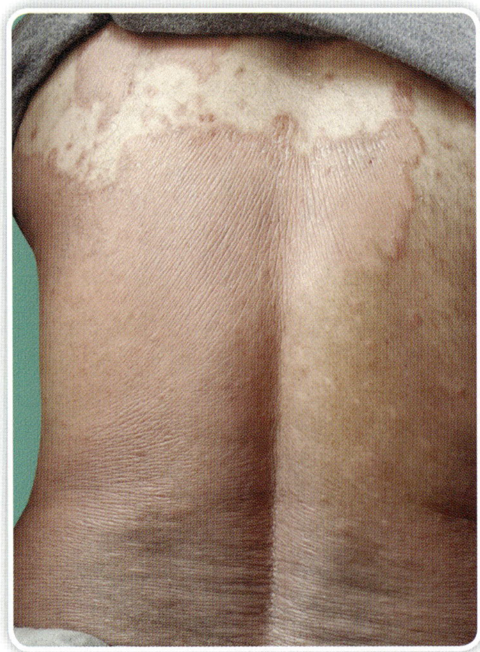

FIG. 8.6: Large irregular extensive plaques of psoriasis over the back of same patient

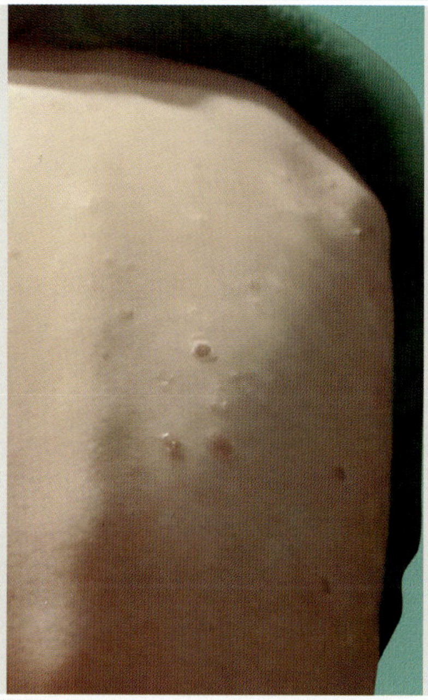

FIG. 8.7: Well-defined psoriatic lesions with postinflammatory hypopigmentation over the back in a male patient

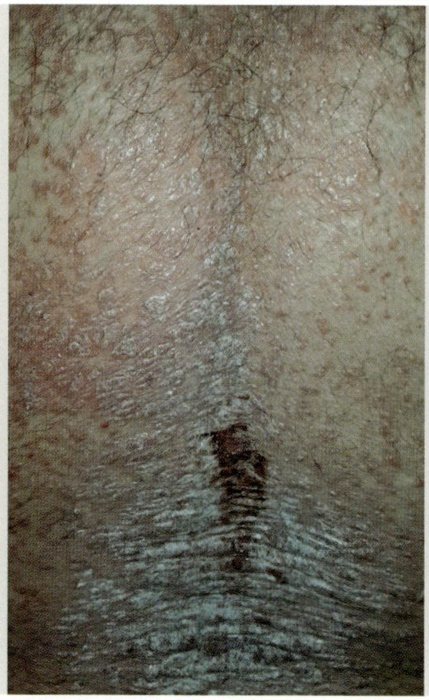

FIG. 8.8: Characteristic psoriatic lesions over the back

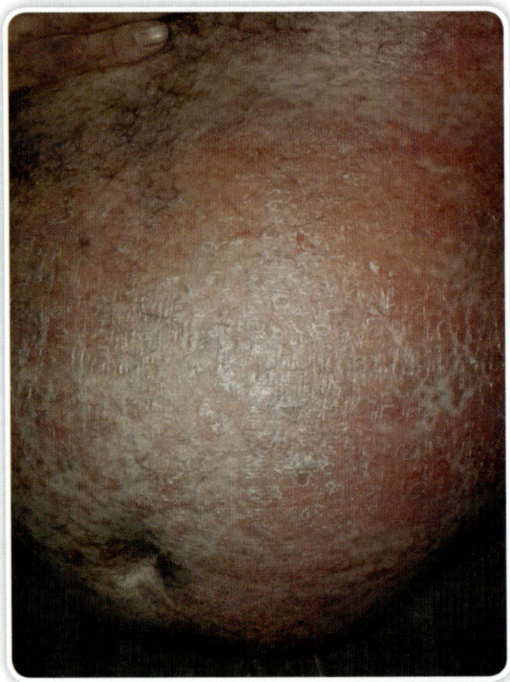

FIG. 8.9: Same patient showing psoriatic lesions over the abdomen

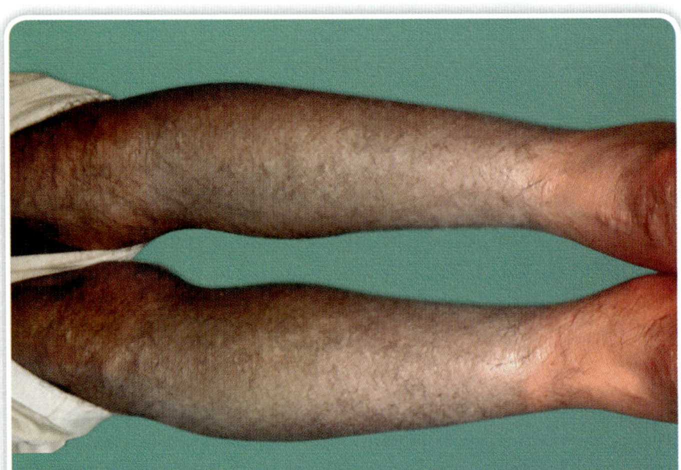

FIG. 8.10: Note large psoriatic plaques over both lower legs. The patient was on topical dithranol therapy with good response

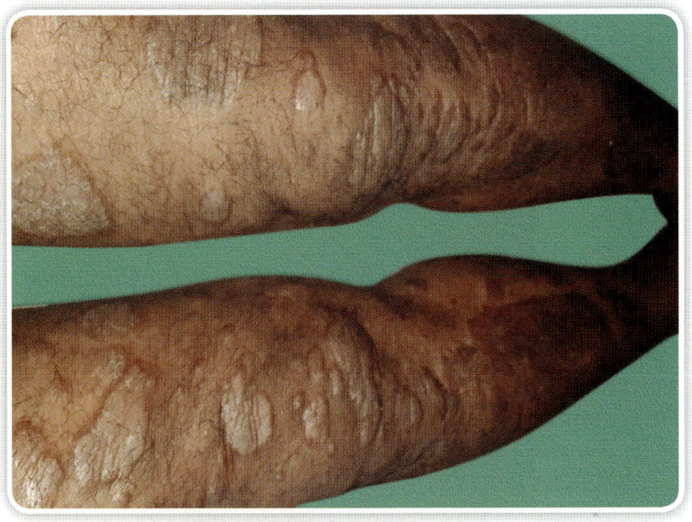

FIG. 8.11: Characteristic well-defined psoriatic plaques over both lower limbs in a middle-aged patient

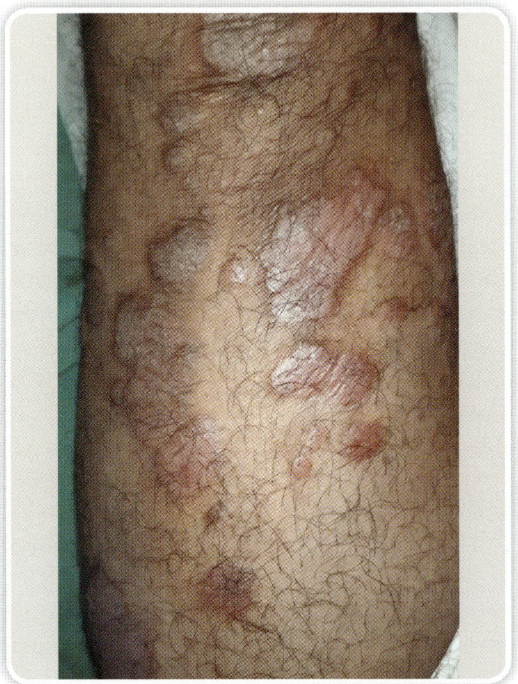

FIG. 8.12: A closer view of psoriatic plaques in the same patient

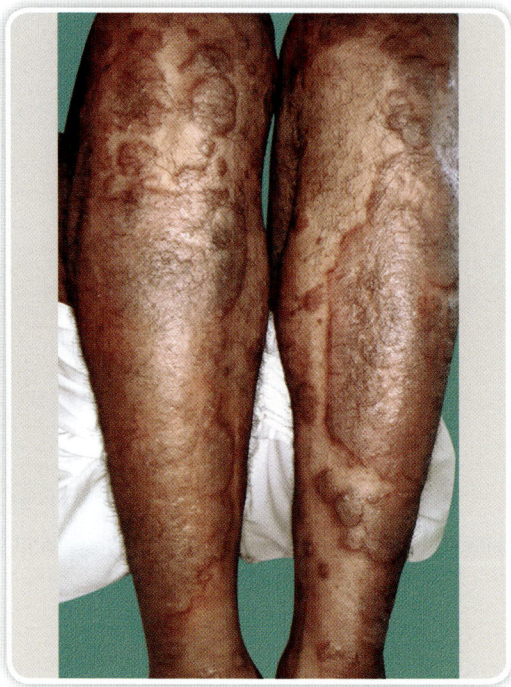

FIG. 8.13: Same patient showing large psoriatic plaques over legs

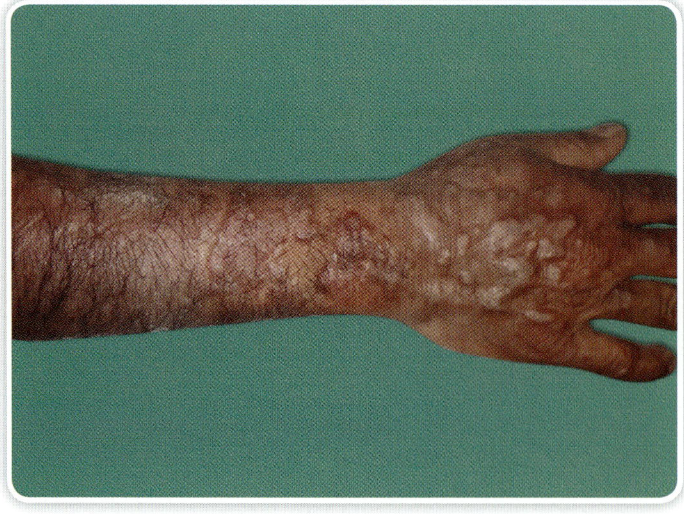

FIG. 8.14: Plaques of psoriasis vulgaris involving the forearm and dorsum of right hand

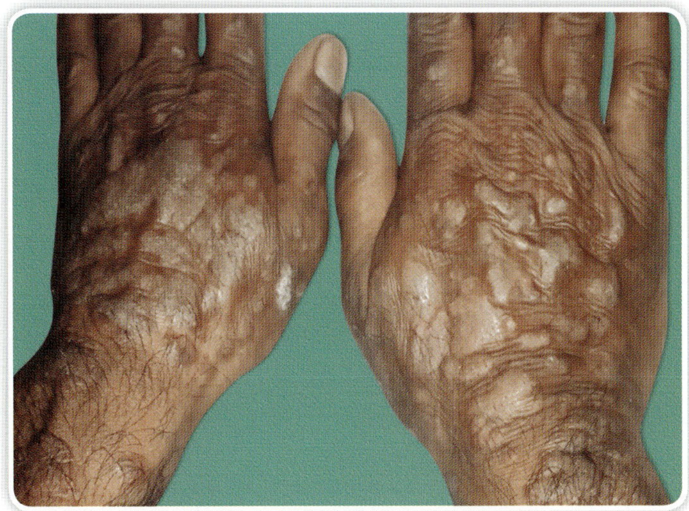

FIG. 8.15: Bilaterally symmetrical plaques of psoriasis over hands. The lesions can be mistaken for plaque type PLE

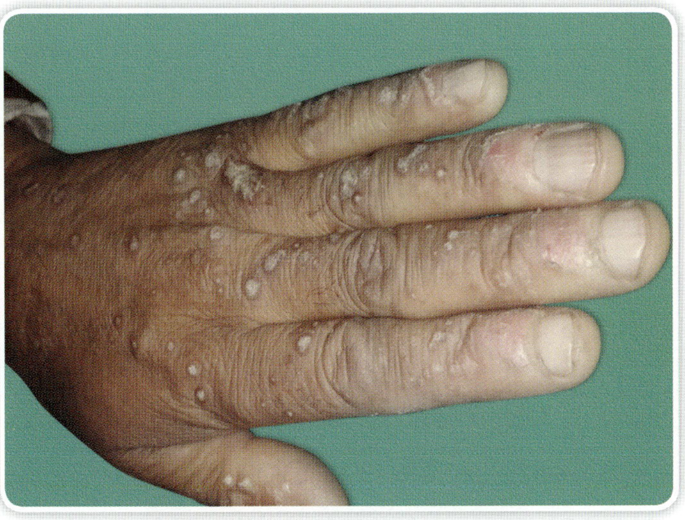

FIG. 8.16: Small psoriatic lesions over the dorsum of left hand. The lesions can be mistaken for perforating dermatosis

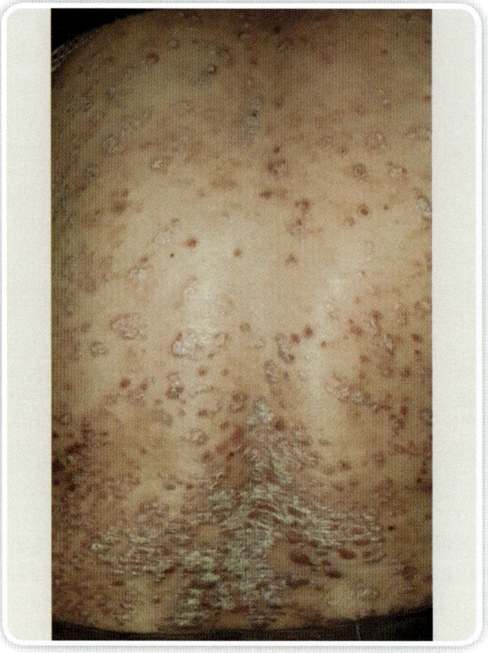

FIG. 8.17: Characteristic plaques of psoriasis over the back

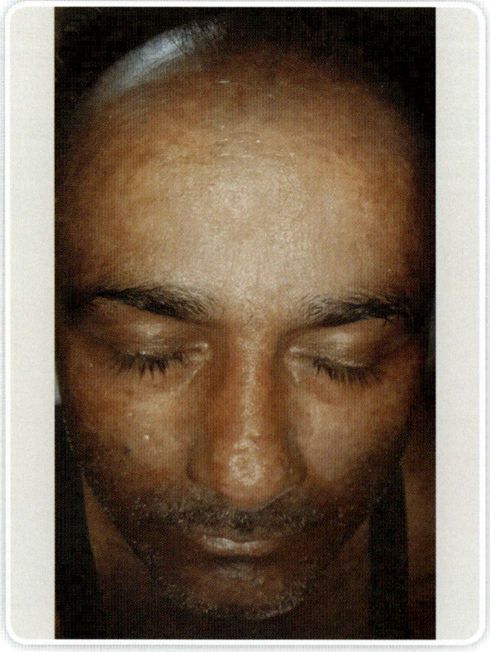

FIG. 8.18: Psoriatic lesions involving the face in a middle-aged patient

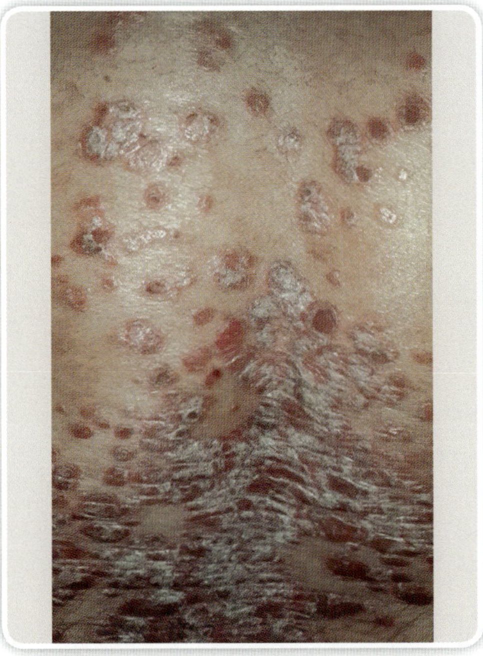

FIG. 8.19: Characteristic plaques of psoriasis with silvery scaling over the back

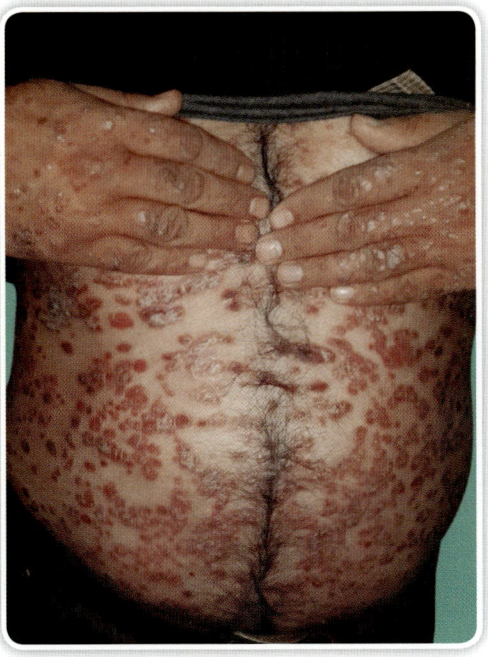

FIG. 8.20: Extensive psoriasis with characteristic lesions over trunk and limbs

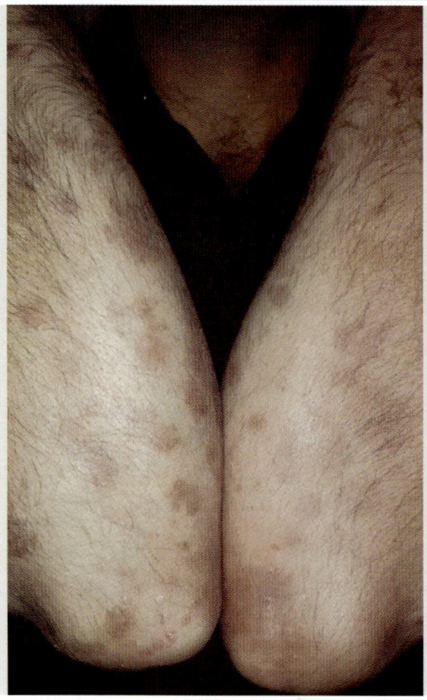

FIG. 8.21: Postinflammatory hyperpigmentation following resolution of psoriatic lesions over upper limbs

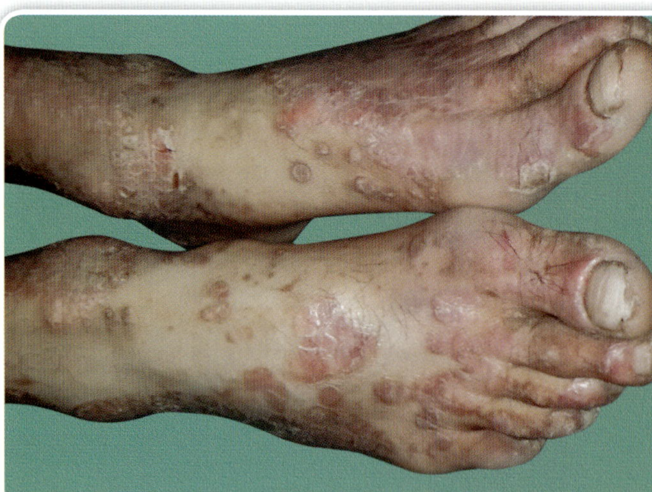

FIG. 8.22: Characteristic plaques of psoriasis over the dorsa of both feet

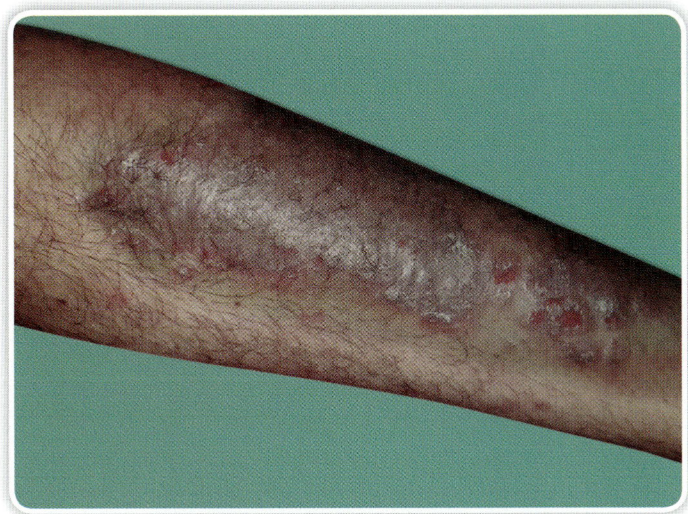

FIG. 8.23: Resolving psoriatic plaque over the leg in a male patient. The patient was on topical dithranol

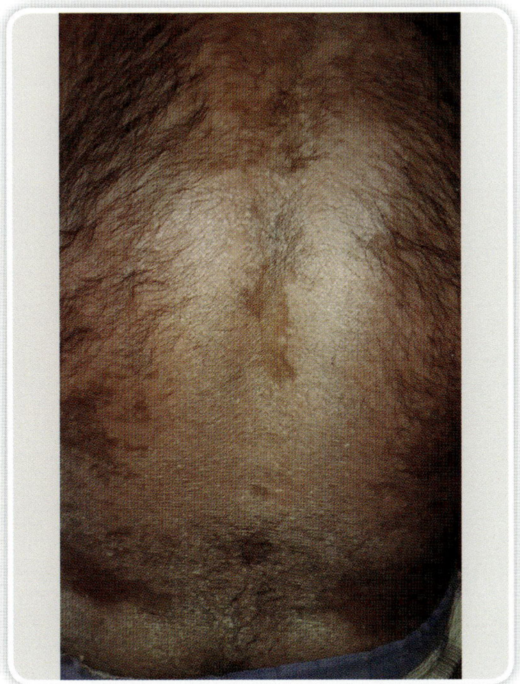

FIG. 8.24: Resolving psoriatic lesions over the back in a male patient

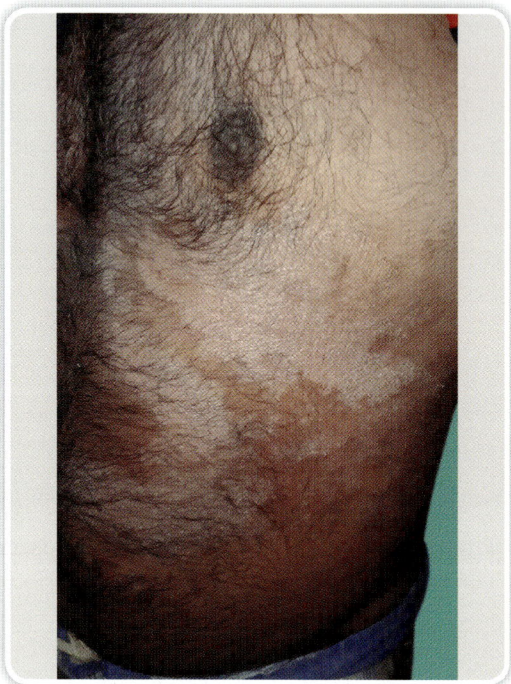

FIG. 8.25: Same patient showing resolving psoriatic lesions over the anterior aspect of trunk

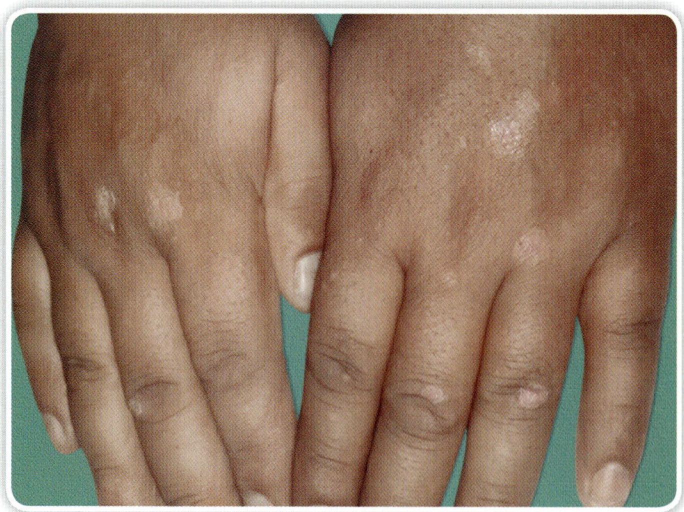

FIG. 8.26: Resolving psoriatic lesions over the dorsa of hands. The lesions can be mistaken for PLE

Flexural or Inverse Psoriasis

Flexural or inverse psoriasis is commonly found in the skin folds, particularly the axillae, submammary regions groin and natal cleft. In this clinical variant of psoriasis, the skin is shiny, red and typically devoid of scales and the plaques are thin. The frequency of flexural psoriasis alone is low, although it may be seen in association with involvement of other parts of the body. It may occur as a primary disorder or as a Koebner phenomenon on top of infective or seborrhoeic intertriginous dermatoses (Figs 8.27 and 8.28).[3]

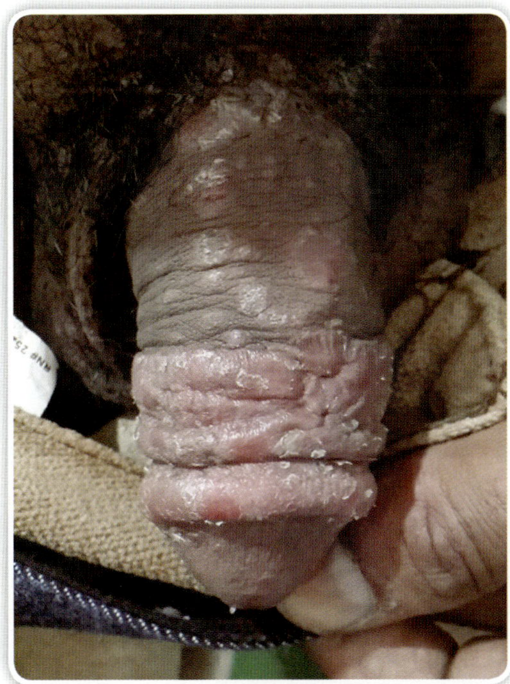

FIG. 8.27: Characteristic lesions of psoriasis involving the penis

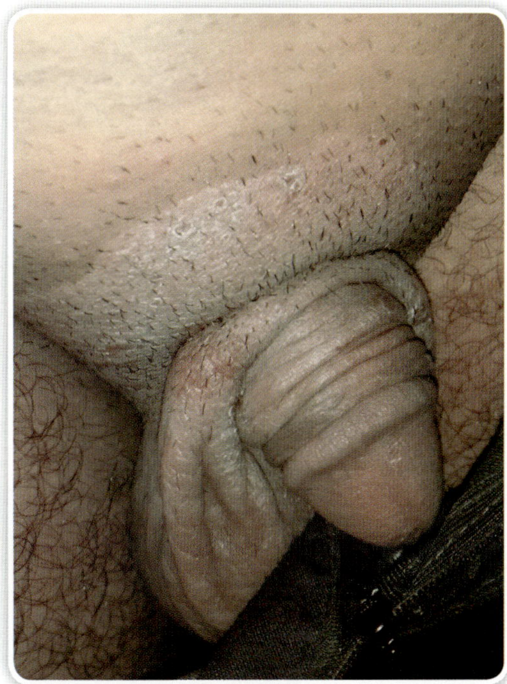

FIG. 8.28: Well-defined psoriatic plaques involving the genital region including groins

Guttate or Eruptive Psoriasis

Guttate or eruptive psoriasis is characterized by lesions that are less than 1 cm in diameter and are found over the upper trunk and proximal extremities. This type of psoriasis typically occurs in children and adolescents and frequently appears following a bacterial or viral infection of the upper airways. The lesions appear suddenly and are self-resolving, clearing within 3–4 weeks. The diagnosis is made chiefly on the nature of scaling, the general distribution and evidence for preceding infections. While the long-term prognosis has not been established, one study concluded that one third of individuals with guttate psoriasis develop classic plaque disease within 10 years (Figs 8.29 to 8.33).[4]

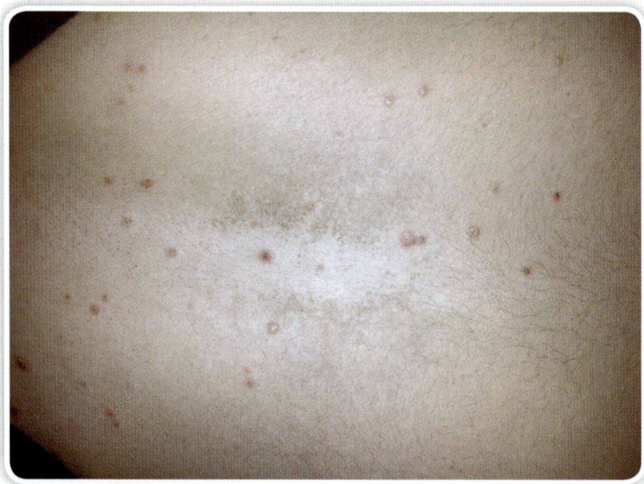

FIG. 8.29: Guttate psoriatic lesions in a young girl. There was a history of preceding sore throat

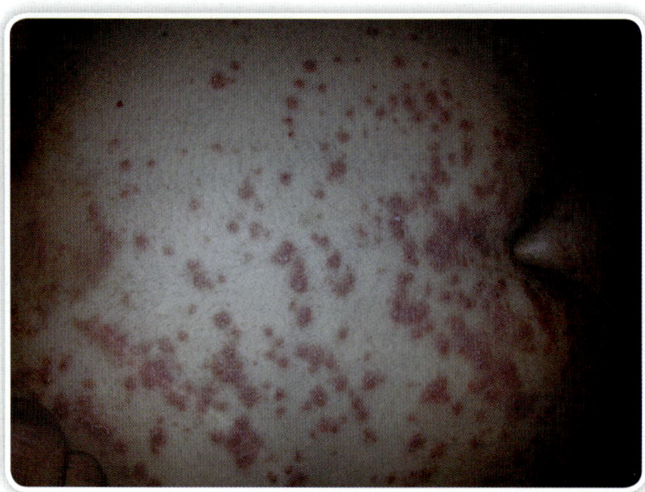

FIG. 8.30: Note the guttate psoriatic lesions superimposed on existing psoriatic lesions in a 30-year-old female precipitated by throat infection

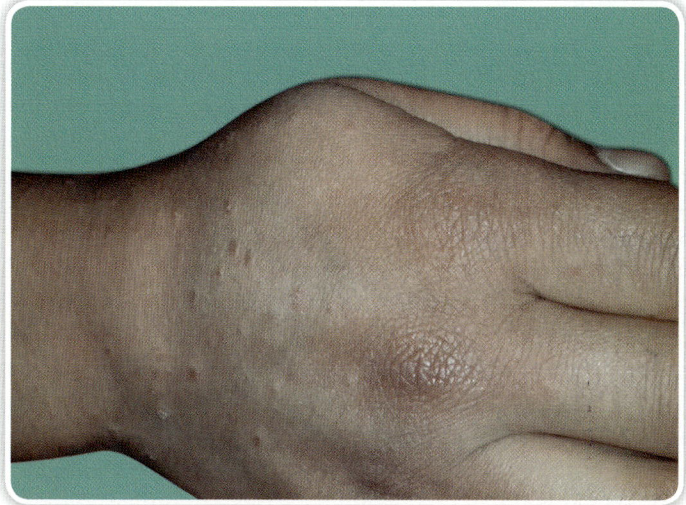

FIG. 8.31: Guttate psoriatic lesions over the dorsum of right hand

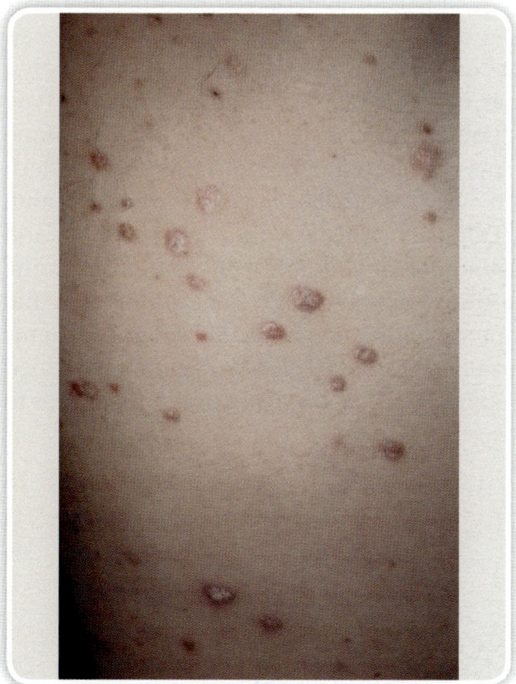

FIG. 8.32: Guttate psoriatic lesions over the trunk in a young male

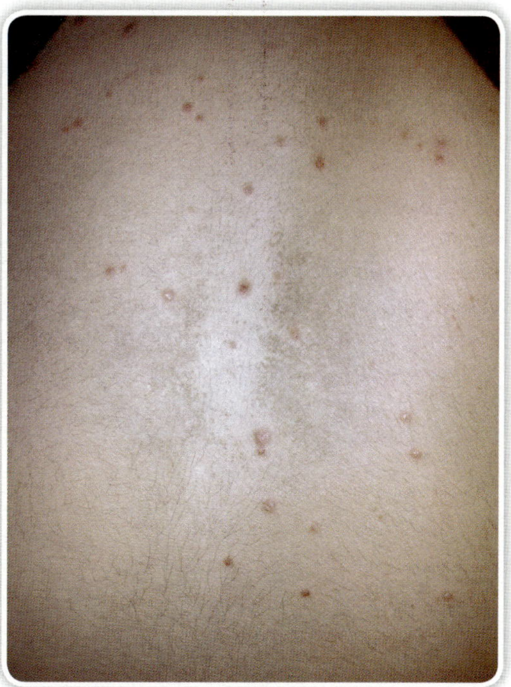

FIG. 8.33: Another patient showing guttate psoriatic lesions over the back

Pustular

Also known as von Zumbusch psoriasis, this is an acute form in which small, monomorphic, sterile pustules develop in painful inflamed skin, involving both the involved as well as uninvolved skin. It is often precipitated by infections and abrupt withdrawal of systemic and potent topical corticosteroids. Many smaller pustules may form on an erythematous base and join up to form a lake of pus. Patients often experience associated weakness, weight loss and episodes of fever that correspond to new outbreaks of pustules.[5]

Palmoplantar

Palmoplantar psoriasis resembles pustular psoriasis and is associated with yellow-brown sterile pustules on the palms and soles. It is predominantly found in women and/or current or previous smokers. Palmoplantar involvement can occur in isolation but often occurs with psoriasis elsewhere on the body. Though only small body surface area is affected but because of the disabling sequelae, this site of involvement carries a definite significance. Palmoplantar involvement can occur in the form of well-defined erythematous scaly plaques or pustular lesions which can present as palmoplantar pustulosis or acrodermatitis continua of hallopeau (Figs 8.34 to 8.38).

Kumar et al. did a comprehensive study on 540 patients having significant palmar and/ or plantar involvement with or without psoriasis elsewhere over the body. Those having extensive psoriasis (>30% BSA) or erythrodermic psoriasis or generalized pustular psoriasis were excluded from the study. Out of total cases, only 15 (2.8%) had pustular lesions, 11 had palmoplantar pustulosis and 4 had acrodermatitis continua of hallopeau. Males outnumbered females and the male to female ratio was similar to that observed in chronic plaque type psoriasis. Most of the patients had involvement of both palms and soles (47.5%) or palms alone (44.3%) while isolated sole (8.1%) involvement was uncommon. The most common pattern of involvement was of plaque type lesions situated over pressure bearing areas on palms and, discrete plaques present randomly over the soles. Extension of lesions onto dorsa of hands and feet and inter digital spaces was also observed. Palmoplantar psoriasis leads to morbidity due to itching, fissuring, difficulty in walking and performing manual tasks. It was thus believed that friction plays a role in localizing the lesions over certain areas on palms and soles in patients with preexisting palmoplantar psoriasis. High prevalence of plantar involvement was ascribed to Indian custom of walking bare foot or wearing open slippers most of the time which leads to frequent minor trauma compared to closed footwear.[6]

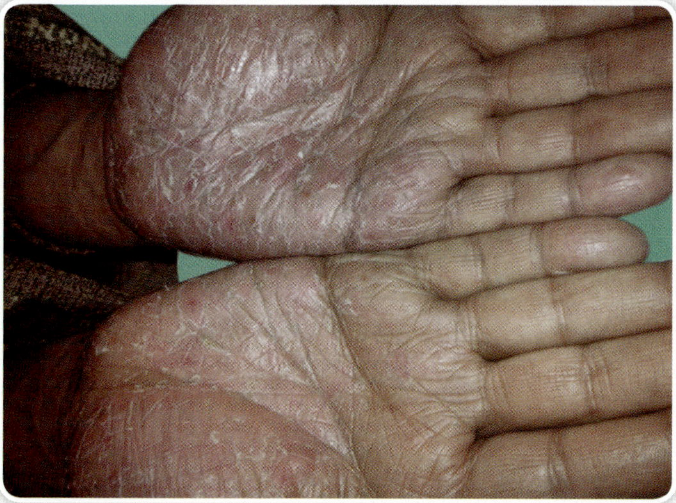

FIG. 8.34: Characteristic lesions of psoriasis involving the palms with sharp demarcation at the wrists.

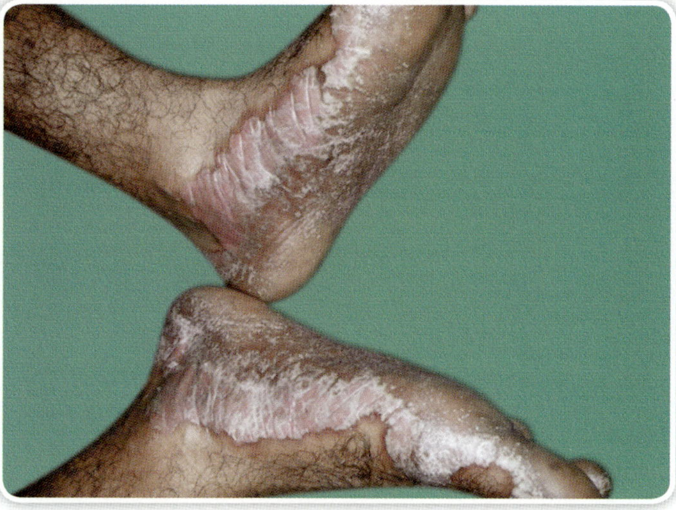

FIG. 8.35: Characteristic plantar lesions of psoriasis in a young male patient.

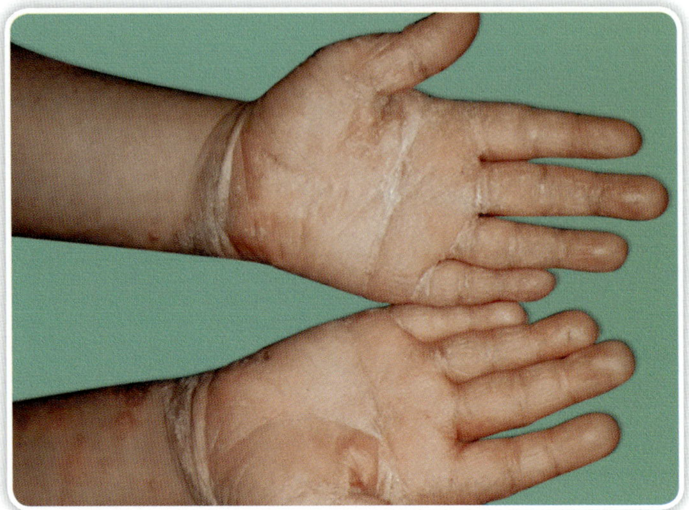

FIG. 8.36: Diffuse involvement of palms in psoriasis. Note few psoriatic lesions over right forearm

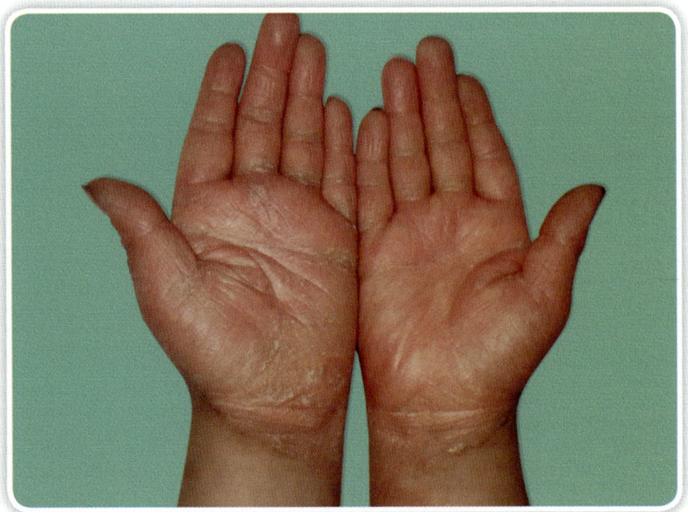

FIG. 8.37: Palmar psoriasis in a young patient. Note the sharp border at the wrist

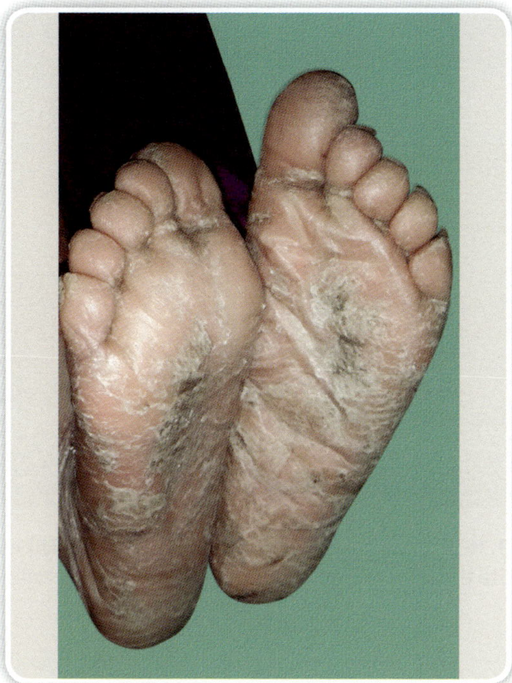

FIG. 8.38: Plantar psoriasis in a 9-year-old girl. Note the characteristic erythema and scaling

Erythrodermic[7,8]

Erythrodermic psoriasis is the clinical variant of psoriasis in which greater than 90% of the body surface area is involved. The skin appears bright red and is covered by superficial fine and loose white scales. This can lead to hypothermia, hypoalbuminemia and high-output cardiac failure. Erythrodermic psoriasis can be life threatening. Psoriasis is an important and common cause of erythroderma. Psoriatic erythroderma can appear de novo or it occurs when chronic plaque type psoriasis leads to extensive involvement (Figs 8.39 to 8.44). Sarkar et al. in an Indian study observed 17 cases of childhood erythroderma over a period of five years suggesting that psoriatic erythroderma is uncommon in children (18% of the total cases) compared to adults. In a recent study by Prakash et al. psoriasis was clinically suspected in 12 of the total 24 patients of erythroderma. Nanda et al. observed erythroderma in 2 (1.8%) out of 112 children with psoriasis seen over nine years (1980–1988) in North India.

Erythrodermic Psoriasis Usually Occurs in Two Contexts

1. In a setting of known, progressively worsening chronic plaque psoriasis.
2. It may be precipitated by infections, tar, drugs, or withdrawal of systemic or potent topical corticosteroids. It is then considered to be part of the spectrum of unstable psoriasis.

Very occasionally, it can be the first presentation of psoriasis.

Erythroderma is a dermatological emergency, which can be fatal and requires urgent inpatient management due to skin failure.

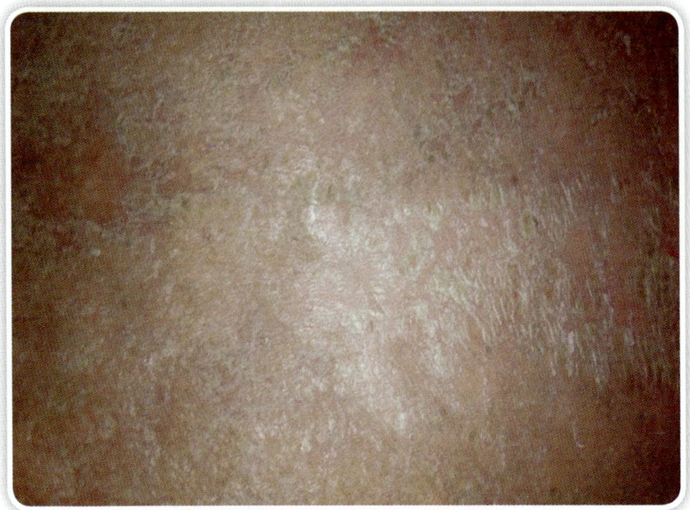

FIG. 8.39: Psoriatic erythroderma in an adult female patient. Note the generalised erythema and superficial scaling

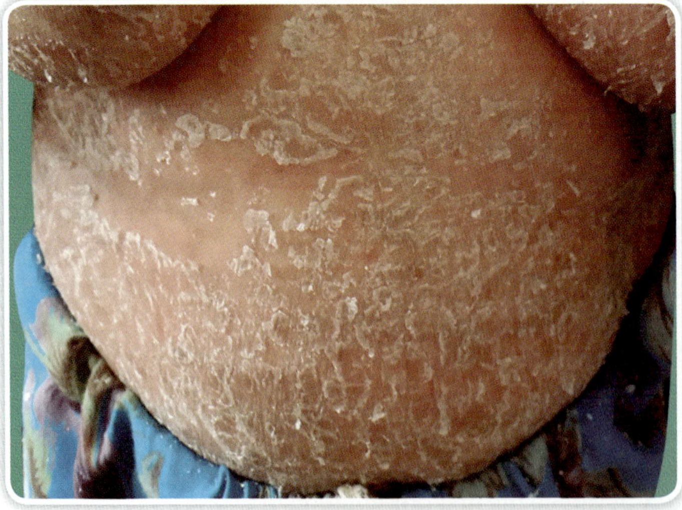

FIG. 8.40: Diffuse erythema with scaling of psoriatic erythroderma in a female

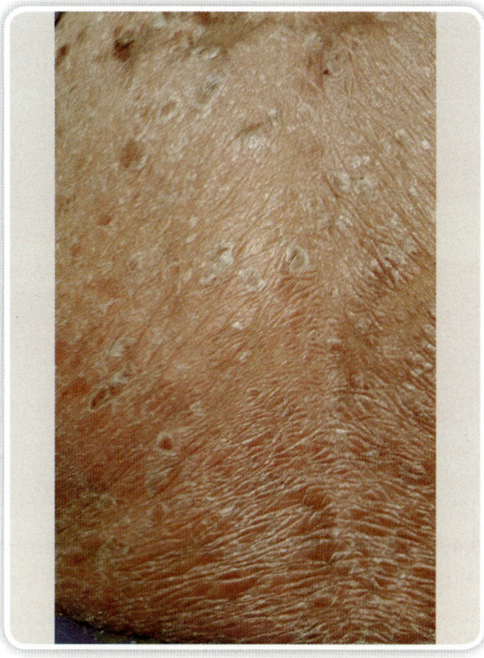

FIG. 8.41: Involvement of back in psoriatic erythroderma in the same patient

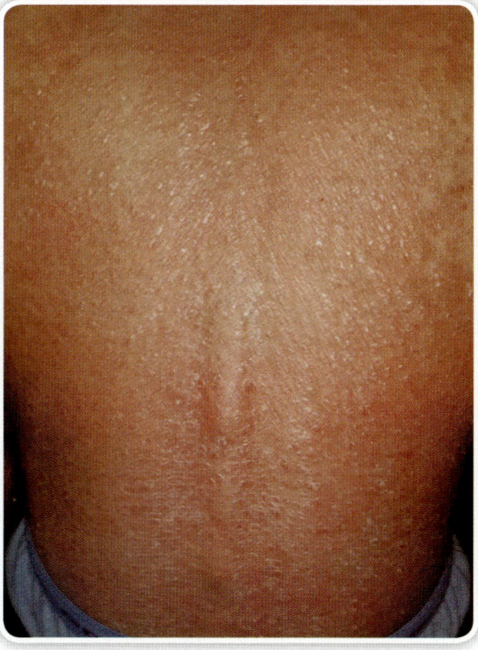

FIG. 8.42: Psoriatic erythroderma in an 18-year-old male patient

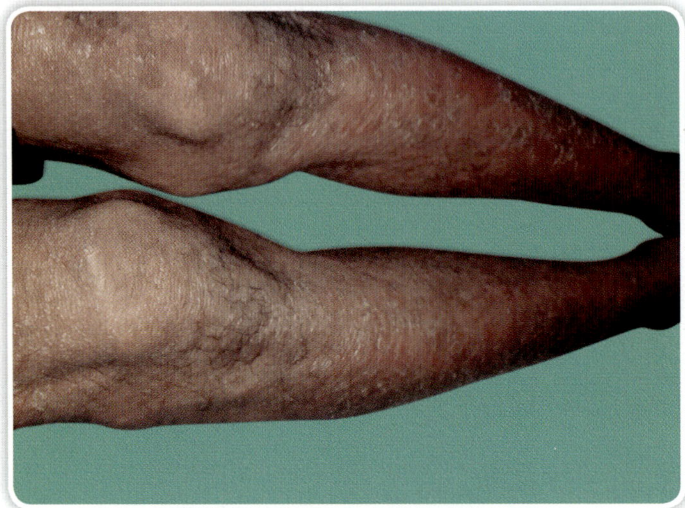

FIG. 8.43: Involvement of lower limbs in the same patient

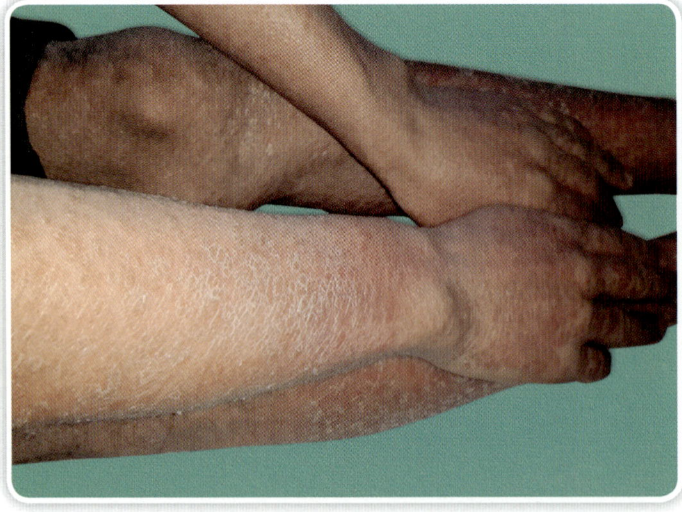

FIG. 8.44: Involvement of both upper and lower limbs in the same patient

Clinical Presentation

In psoriatic erythroderma, the whole skin is red and hot with the dermatological characteristics of psoriasis being often lost. The scales are usually finer and flakier than the classic silvery, coarse scales of psoriasis. Itching and burning pain are usual and may be severe. There is associated history of skin tenderness, fever, malaise, decreased appetite, constipation and oliguria. The patient is often systemically unwell.

Differential Diagnosis

Psoriatic erythroderma has to be distinguished from other causes of erythroderma, viz;

1. Eczema (contact, atopic, seborrhoeic).
2. Lymphoma, particularly Sézary syndrome.
3. Psoriasiform drug eruptions: Due to allopurinol, gold, isoniazid, phenytoin, sulphonamides, sulphonylureas.
4. Pityriasis rubra pilaris.
5. Ichthyosiform erythroderma.

Investigations

- The diagnosis is mainly clinical, based on the history and presentation
- Where the cause of the erythroderma is known to be psoriasis, investigations should be done to look for the presence of complications and their extent. So, in addition to the baseline investigations (CBC, urine examination, KFT, LFT) inflammatory markers and blood cultures are taken to look for renal failure, anemia, hypoalbuminaemia and infection. Additionally, efforts should be made to identify any triggers.

Associated diseases and precipitants are:

- Infections
- Hypocalcemia
- Oral (or potent topical) corticosteroid withdrawal
- Application of strong coal tar preparations
- Drug-induced, eg; lithium, antimalarials, interleukin-2.

Management

Following emergency admission, management requires skilled nursing care and includes:

- Bed rest in a warm ambient temperature (30–32°C)
- Emollients and cool wet dressings
- Treatment of complications
- Nutritional support.

There is a dearth of high-quality evidence on which to base treatment decisions:

- Topical tar therapy and phototherapy should be avoided in the early phases of treatment
- Retinoids have also been reported to induce this condition
- Corticosteroid treatment is tricky: Subsequent withdrawal may worsen the clinical state but, sometimes, this is the only effective treatment for the acute episode

- Ciclosporin and infliximab are the most rapid-acting agents, with acitretin and methotrexate the slower-acting first-line choices
- Combination therapy may be more effective but this remains unproven.

Complications

The complications of psoriatic erythroderma include:
- Dehydration
- Impaired thermoregulation and hypothermia
- Cardiac failure
- Overwhelming infection
- Protein loss and edema
- Anemia (loss of iron, vitamin B12 and folate)
- Lymphadenopathy (dermatopathic)
- Rarely death.

Prognosis

The prognosis is variable: Where there is preexisting, extensive plaque psoriasis, treatment is usually well tolerated and the prognosis is good; however, with unstable psoriasis, the course is often prolonged, relapses are frequent and there is an associated mortality.

Prevention

There are no specific preventive measures other than optimising the management of pre-existing psoriasis and avoiding precipitating factors.[9,10]

Points to Remember

- Psoriasis has a number of clinical variants that differ in severity, location, longevity, shape, pattern, cause and treatment. The different types of psoriasis are fairly distinct. Patients may experience more than one type at the same time
- The prognosis is variable where there is preexisting, extensive-plaque psoriasis, treatment is usually well-tolerated and the prognosis is good; however, with unstable psoriasis, the course is often prolonged, relapses are frequent and there is an associated mortality
- Chronic plaque psoriasis is the most common type

Scalp

Scalp psoriasis is characterized by very-thick plaques on the scalp and along the hair margin, the plaques becoming thicker and crusted as the disease develops. The whole scalp may be diffusely involved, or multiple discrete plaques of varying size may be seen. While the scalp is the major area involved, in some cases the lesions may extend to the forehead, neck, ear and retroauricular areas. It is always encouraging for patients to know that scalp psoriasis does not cause alopecia. A morphological entity consisting of plaques of asbestos-like scaling, firmly adherent to the scalp and associated hair, has been termed pityriasis amiantacea, which may result in cicatricial alopecia sometimes. It is a nonspecific reaction pattern, which may be seen in other scaling scalp conditions such as seborrhoeic dermatitis (Figs 8.45 to 8.48).

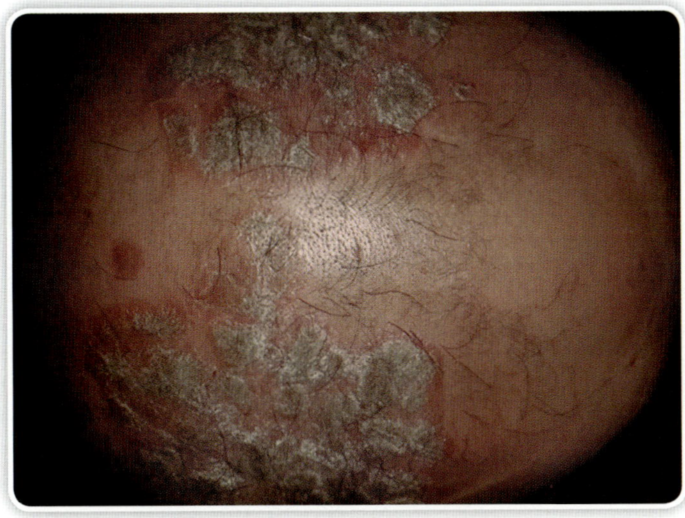

FIG. 8.45: Characteristic psoriatic plaques involving the scalp in a middle aged male.

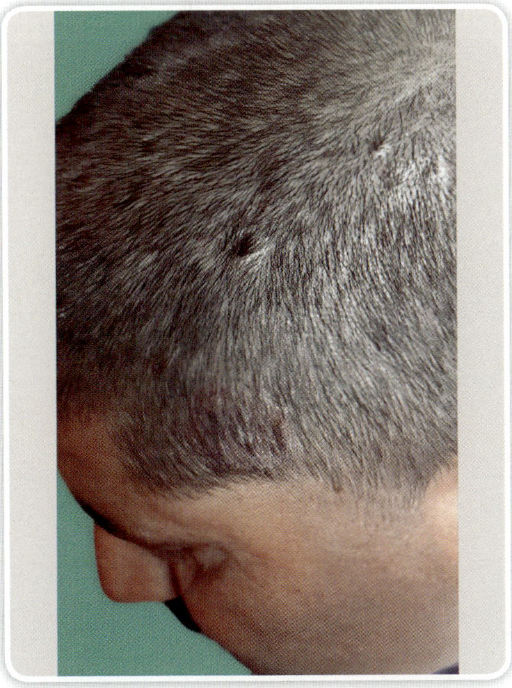

FIG. 8.46: Multiple well-defined plaques of psoriasis over scalp in a middle-aged male

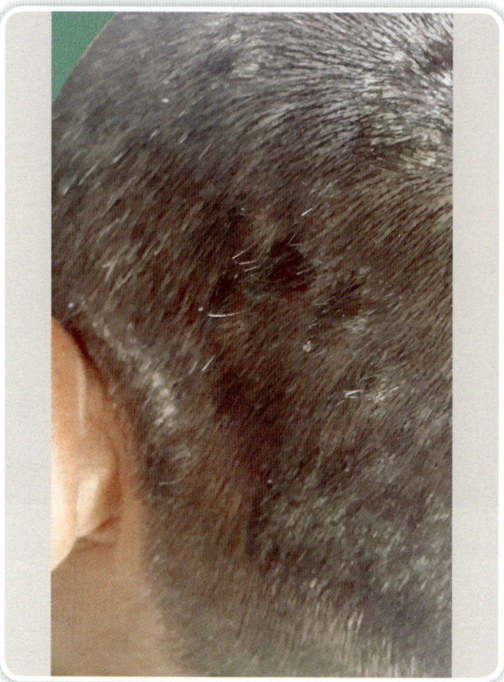

FIG. 8.47: Same patient showing multiple psoriatic plaques over the posterior aspect of scalp

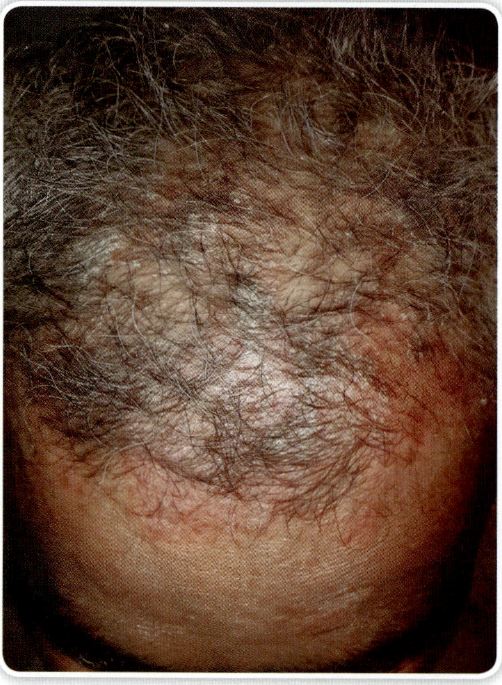

FIG. 8.48: Erythematous scaly plaques of psoriasis involving scalp in a male patient

Topical Treatments for Scalp Psoriasis

Scalp psoriasis can be intractable and resistant to therapy. The first line of defense against scalp psoriasis is tar containing shampoos. The two medications which are approved by FDA for the treatment of scalp psoriasis include:

Salicylic Acid and Coal Tar

Tar-containing shampoos should be the first approach and shampooing should be carried out daily if necessary. Coal tar containing lotions or gels may be added, to be applied at night and shampooed out the following morning. Prescription products for scalp psoriasis may contain higher concentrations of salicylic acid, coal tar, or both as well as other FDA-approved medications. Other drugs that are used in scalp psoriasis and have been found to be effective in various studies are as follows:

- Anthralin
- Corticosteroid scalp lotions, gels and foams
- Antimicrobials, which are used to treat bacterial or yeast infections associated with scalp psoriasis
- Calcipotriene, a vitamin D derivative
- Calcipotriene and betamethasone dipropionate (a potent steroid)
- Tazarotene, a vitamin A derivative.[11]

Nail Psoriasis

Psoriatic nail disease is frequently seen in patients, with approximately 50% of the fingernails and 35% of the toenails being affected; the average nail involvement being 25–50%. The changes range from minor alterations in the nail plate to severe defects and include pitting, onycholysis (nail plate separations), oil spots (orange-yellow subungual discoloration), dystrophy and splinter hemorrhages. Nail involvement is common in psoriasis and can be the initial and the only site of involvement in some patients. Morphology of nail changes depends on whether nail matrix, nail bed or hyponychium has been affected. Nail involvement is more common in those who have concurrent psoriatic arthritis. Bedi in an Indian study noted nail changes in 74% of total patients while isolated nail affliction was seen in 6% of cases. Various nail changes observed in descending order of frequency were pitting, thickening of nail plate, partial onycholysis, subungual hyperkeratosis, yellow-brown discoloration, paronychia and complete onycholysis (Figs 8.49 to 8.59).[12,13]

Kaur et al. in a study observed nail changes in 167 psoriasis patients over a period of five years. Of the total cases, 3% had isolated nail involvement. Pitting was the most common nail change, followed by onycholysis, discoloration, subungual hyperkeratosis, longitudinal ridging and thickening of the nail plate. Pits were present in irregular pattern in 90% cases while in rest 10% they were arranged in transverse or longitudinal lines. Two third of their subjects did not have nail fold involvement. While one-third cases who had proximal and/or lateral nail fold involvement, larger body surface area was involved and also a significantly higher mean number of nail changes were present per subject. Ghosal et al. in an another Indian study observed nail involvement in 100 psoriasis patients. Finger nails were involved in

32% and toe nails in 24% cases. Pitting and subungual hyperkeratosis were the most common finger and toe nail changes noted in 65% and 33% cases, respectively. Nail changes were more common in those with joint pain (73%) compared to those who had no joint complaints (30%) and odds ratio was 6.6. They also noted significant association of nail changes with Koebner phenomenon.[14,15]

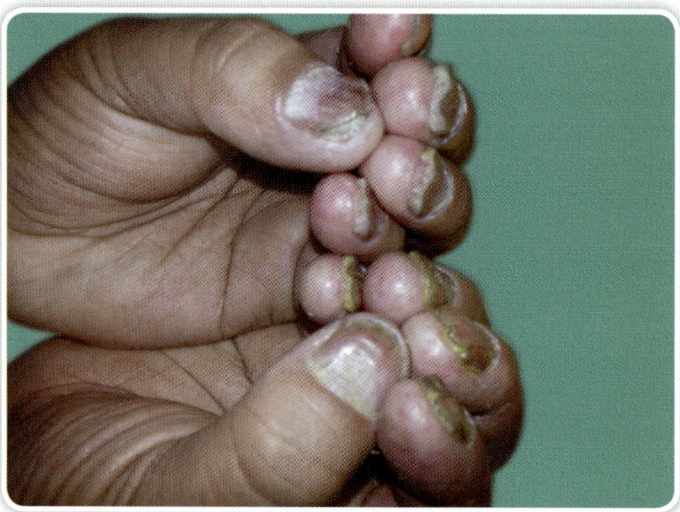

FIG. 8.49: Note the discoloration, SUHK, pitting and Beau's lines in nails affected by psoriasis

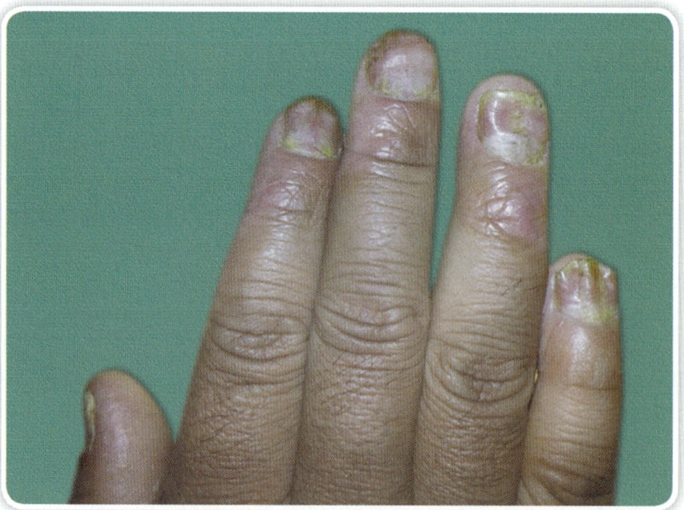

FIG. 8.50: Note the discoloration, pitting, distal onycholysis and crumbling of the nail plates along with involvement of the proximal nail folds

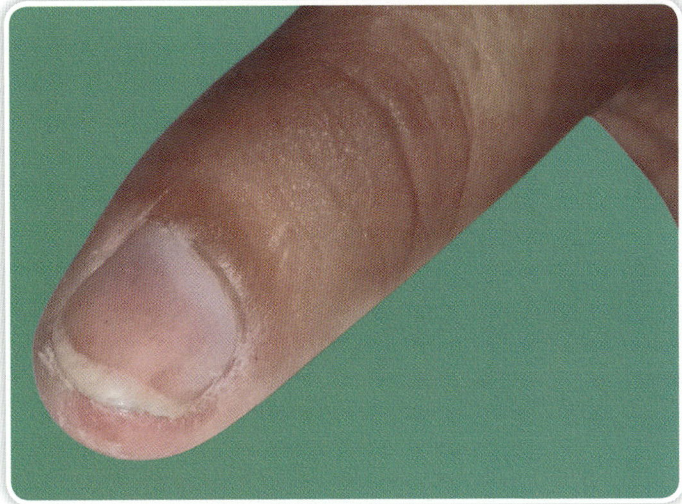

FIG. 8.51: Distal onycholysis in a patient of psoriasis with isolated thumb nail involvement

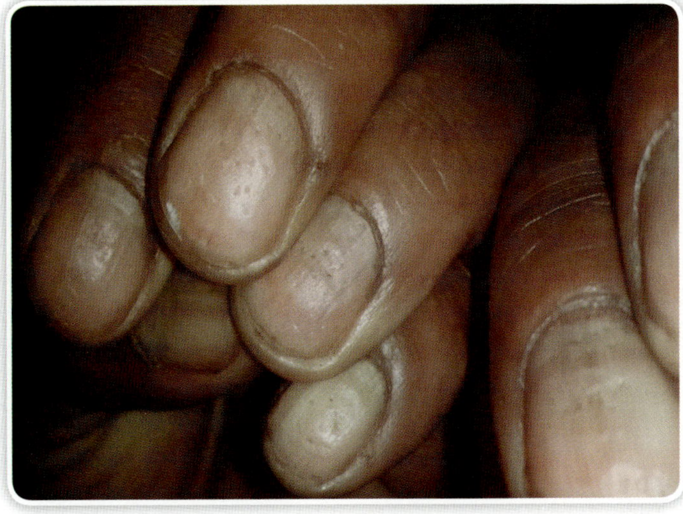

FIG. 8.52: Coarse pitting also known as thimble pitting in multiple psoriatic nails

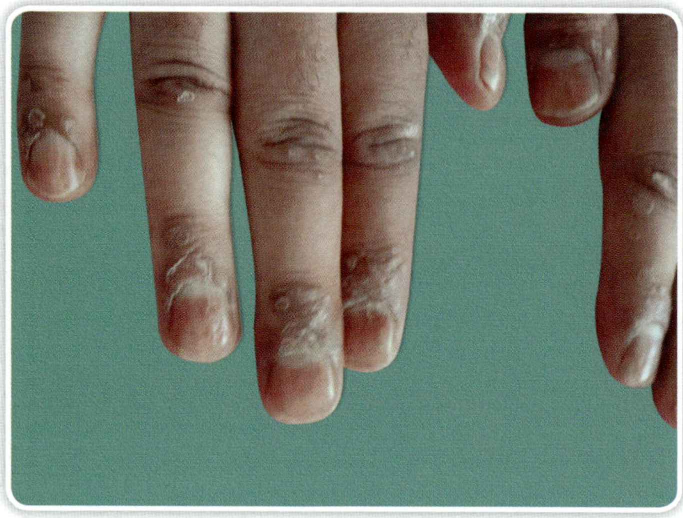

FIG. 8.53: Involvement of nails and terminal interphalangeal joints with psoriatic lesions

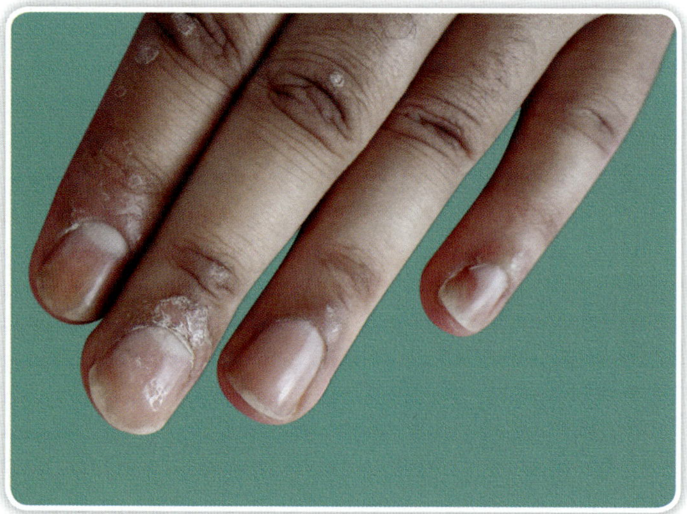

FIG. 8.54: A closer view of nail changes especially pitting in the same patient

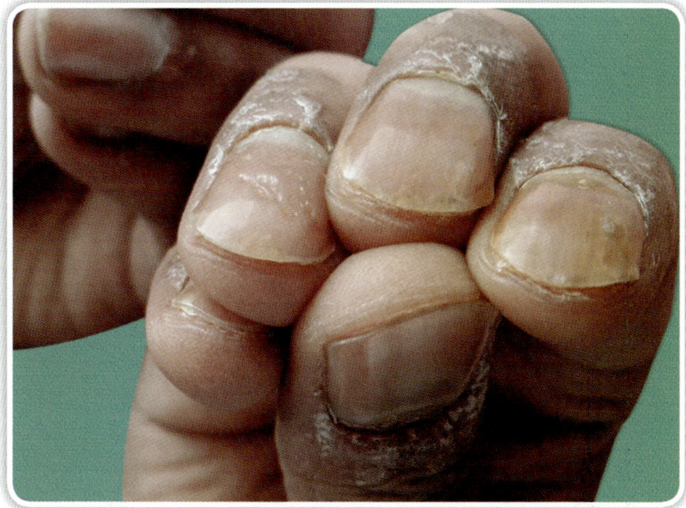

FIG. 8.55: Pitting, distal onycholysis and nail fold involvement in psoriasis

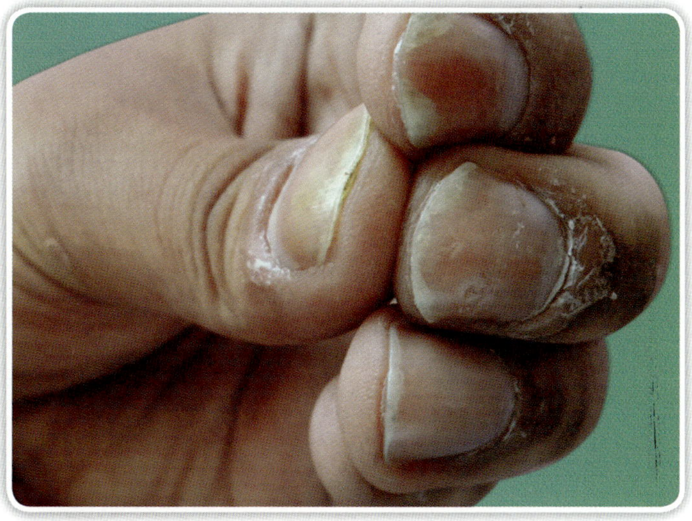

FIG. 8.56: A closer view of nail changes in the same patient

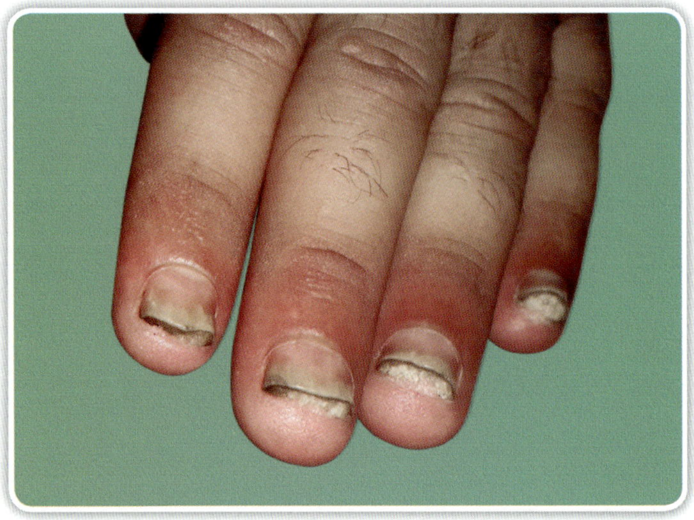

FIG. 8.57: Subungual hyperkeratosis and distal onycholysis of multiple nails in psoriasis

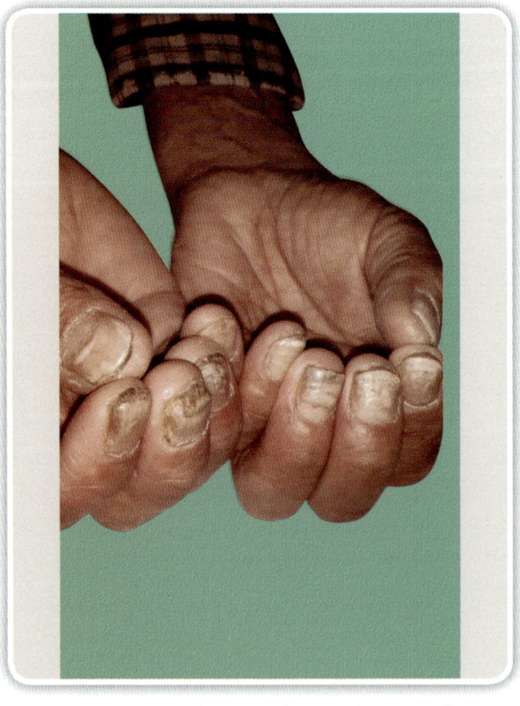

FIG. 8.58: Psoriatic nail dystrophy involving multiple nails

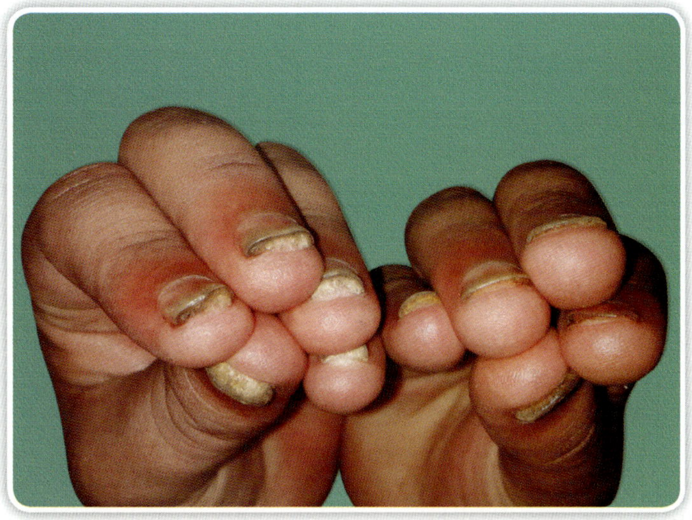

FIG. 8.59: Subungual hyperkeratosis and distal onycholysis of multiple nails in psoriasis

Nail Psoriasis Severity Index

Nail psoriasis severity index (NAPSI) is a numeric, reproducible, objective and simple tool for evaluation of nail psoriasis. This scale is used to evaluate the severity of nail-bed psoriasis and nail-matrix psoriasis by area of involvement in the nail unit. NAPSI is used to assign a score to each nail for nail-bed and nail-matrix psoriasis. In NAPSI, the nail plate is divided into quadrants by imaginary longitudinal and horizontal lines. The nail plate is assessed for nail-matrix psoriasis by the presence of any features of nail-matrix psoriasis, including nail pitting, leukonychia, red spots in the lunula and crumbling in each quadrant of the nail. The nail-bed psoriasis is assessed by the presence of any features of nail-bed psoriasis, including onycholysis, oil drop (salmon patch), splinter hemmorhages and nail-bed hyperkeratosis in each quadrant of the nail.

Scoring

The score is 0 if the findings are not present, 1 if they are present in 1 quadrant of the nail, 2 if present in 2 quadrants of a nail, 3 if present in 3 quadrants of a nail and 4 if present in 4 quadrants of a nail. Thus each nail has a matrix score (0–4) and a nail-bed score (0–4) and the total nail score is the sum of the 2 individual scores. The sum of the total score of all involved fingernails is the total NAPSI score for that patient at that time.[16,17]

If a more sensitive scale is needed, the nail can be given a separate score for all 8 features in each quadrant. The resulting score is a 0–32 scale for the nail.

Modified NAPSI

In a recent report by Mukai et al. NAPSI scores were evaluated in psoriatic patients using acitretin and it was concluded that the method was easy and rapid in measuring the improvement with treatment; however, it did not quantify the existing lesions and might not detect small changes. In 2007, a modified NAPSI (mNAPSI) was proposed by Cassell et al. in order to increase the sensitivity of NAPSI, using a qualitative gradation of severity for each parameter from 0 to 3 in each quadrant. Although it can be time consuming and impractical for the clinicians in an outpatient clinic, modified NAPSI demonstrates excellent interrater reliability and validity in the assessment of psoriatic nail disease. Digital photography might be an easy and convenient method for monitoring the progression of the nail involvement during the treatment.[18]

Treatment options for nail psoriasis.

There are numerous treatment modalities for nail psoriasis but there is little information concerning their effectiveness and safety. Treatments include topical, intramatrix steroid injections, systemic and combination therapies.

Topical treatments: Various studies have demonstrated that the vitamin-D derivative tacalcitol ointment obtains a significant improvement in all nail parameters, both of the matrix and of the bed. Clobetasol nail lacquer; 5-fluorouracil, calcipotriol plus betamethasone dipropionate ointment are also reported to be effective.

Systemic treatments: Low-dose methotrexate and cyclosporine have been tried with varying results. Biologicals especially efalizumab and infliximab have also been reported to be effective.

Intralesional steroid injections.[19,20] These are the treatment of choice for limited nail involvement.

Points to Remember

- Nail changes are observed in 25–50% of patients with psoriasis
- NAPSI is a numeric, reproducible, objective and simple tool for evaluation of nail psoriasis. This scale is used to evaluate the severity of nail-bed psoriasis and nail-matrix psoriasis by area of involvement in the nail unit
- Nail changes are more common in those with psoriatic arthritis and those with koebnerisation

Acral Psoriasis

Recently an unusual chronic dermatosis, considered a new clinical entity and closely resembling psoriasis, has been described in the literature under the term psoriasiform acral dermatitis (PAD). It is characterized by cutaneous involvement of the digits without nail dystrophy. The term PAD was coined by Zaias in 1980 to describe a distinctive psoriasiform dermatitis selectively localized on the distal phalanges of the fingers and associated with a remarkable shortening of the nail bed (Fig. 8.60). In the last few years only 8 patients affected by this unusual chronic dermatosis have been reported in the literature. Seven of these patients were children under 10 years of age. In 1999, Zaias N et al. described PAD in 3 children affected by psoriasis followed up until then and concluded their report with an open question as to whether PAD was a distinctive entity or just a clinical manifestation of psoriasis in children.

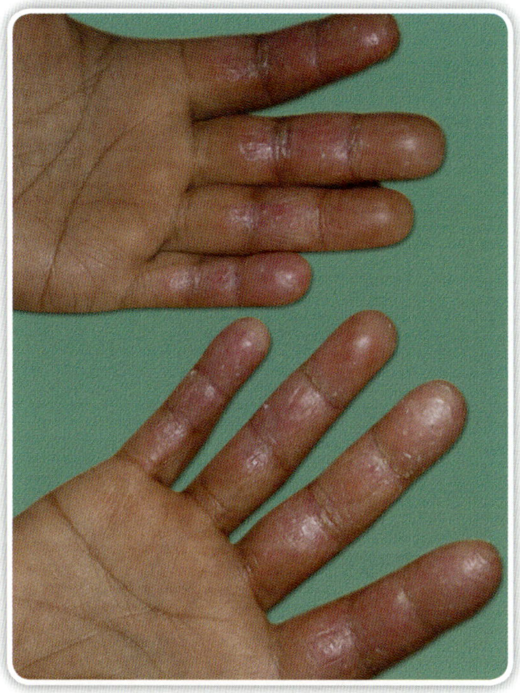

FIG. 8.60: Characteristic acral involvement in acral psoriasis (PAD)

In the latter situation the most appropriate term to define this entity would be "psoriatic acral dermatitis". PAD being a particular variety of acral psoriasis in childhood can be isolated or associated with typical lesions of psoriasis in other cutaneous areas (Fig. 8.60).[21,22]

Seborrheic

Seborrheic psoriasis is a condition whereby seborrheic dermatitis and psoriasis coexist. In many cases, the seborrheic dermatitis leads to psoriasis in the same areas. There tends to be less silvery scaling than psoriasis and more yellowish, greasy scales. Sebopsoriasis tends to localize to the scalp, face and anterior chest in a similar pattern to that seen in seborrheic dermatitis. But sebo-psoriasis has a deeper red color, more defined margins and a thicker scale than typically seen in seborrhoeic dermatitis alone. It is also less likely to clear up with anti-dandruff shampoo (Figs 8.61 to 8.64).[23]

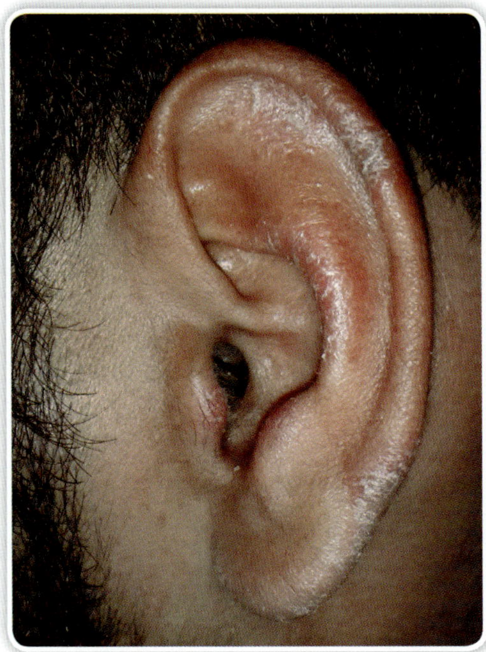

FIG. 8.61: Involvement of pinna with external auditory canal in a patient of sebopsoriasis

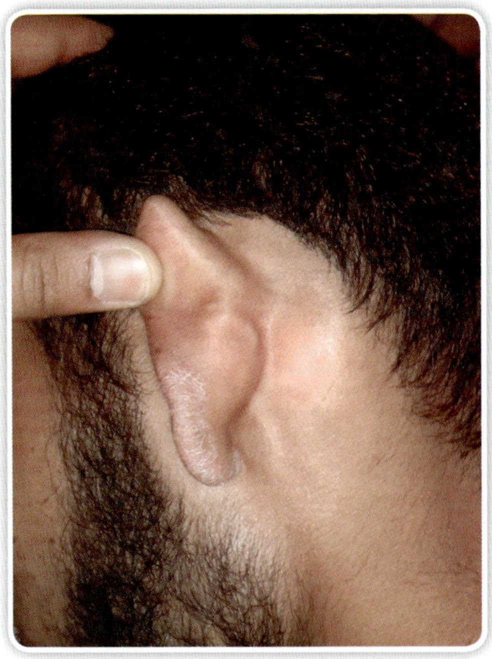

FIG. 8.62: Involvement of retroauricular groove with ear lobule in sebopsoriasis

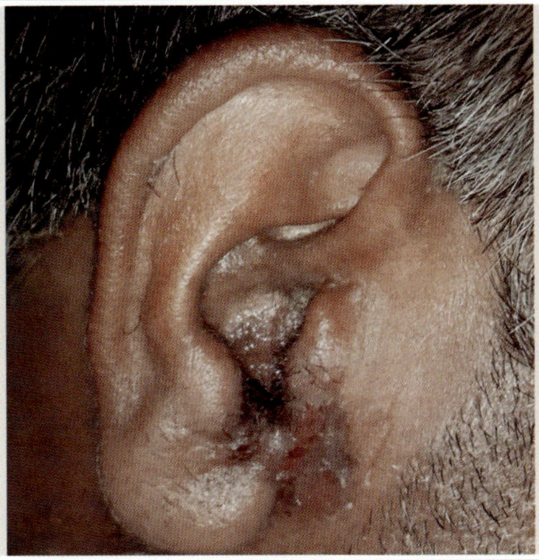

FIG. 8.63: Involvement of external auditory canal with a psoriatic plaque in the preauricular region

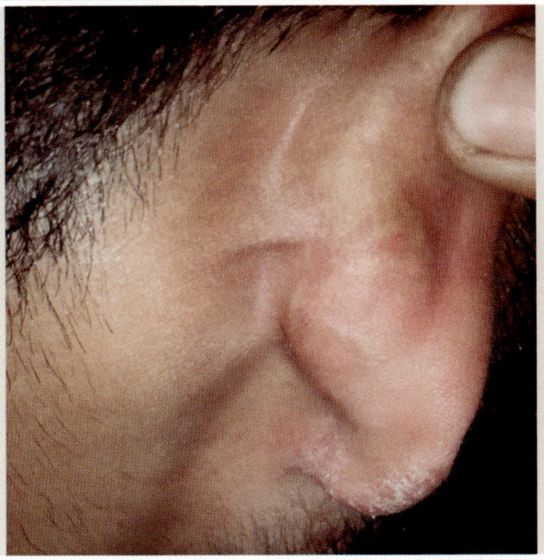

FIG. 8.64: Characteristic plaque of psoriasis involving the ear lobule and retroauricular groove of right side in a male patient

Rupioid, Elephantine and Ostraceous Psoriasis

These rare variants of psoriasis are characterized by plaques with gross hyperkeratosis. Rupioid psoriasis refers to limpet-like cone-shaped lesions. The term elephantine psoriasis is used to describe unusual but persistent thick scaling plaques that usually occur on the back and limbs. Ostraceous psoriasis is characterised by ring-like hyperkeratotic lesions with a concave surface resembling an oyster shell (Figs 8.65 to 8.73).[24]

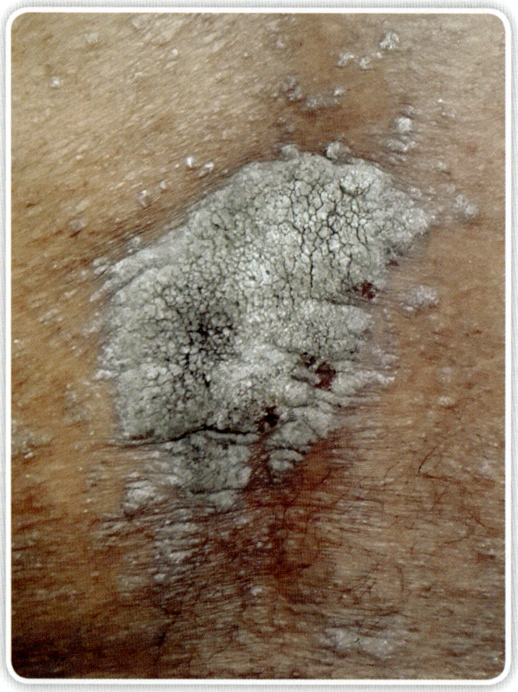

FIG. 8.65: A plaque of rupioid psoriasis involving the back in a 62-year-old male patient. The patient was on NB-UVB therapy

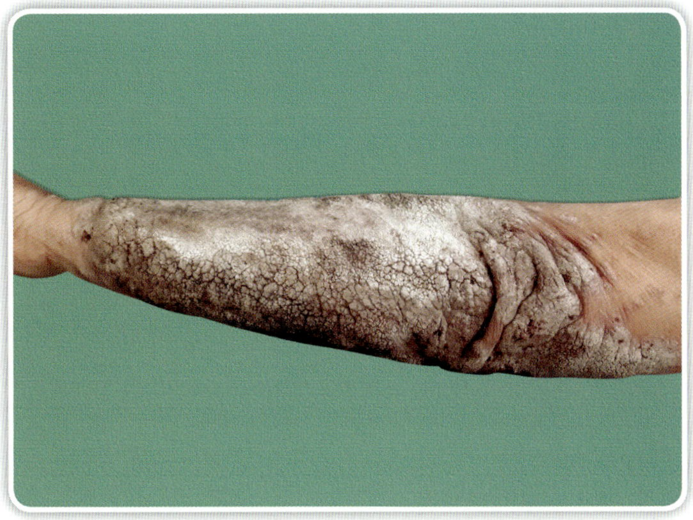

FIG. 8.66: Same patient showing rupioid psoriatic plaques involving the left forearm and arm

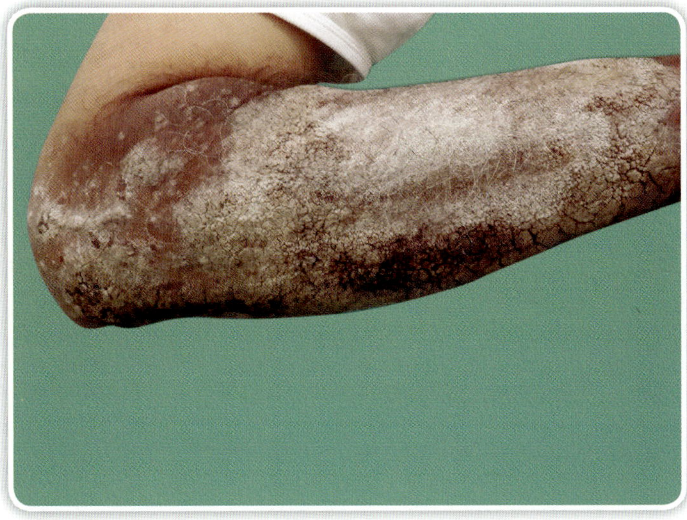

FIG. 8.67: Same patient showing rupioid psoriatic plaques involving the right forearm

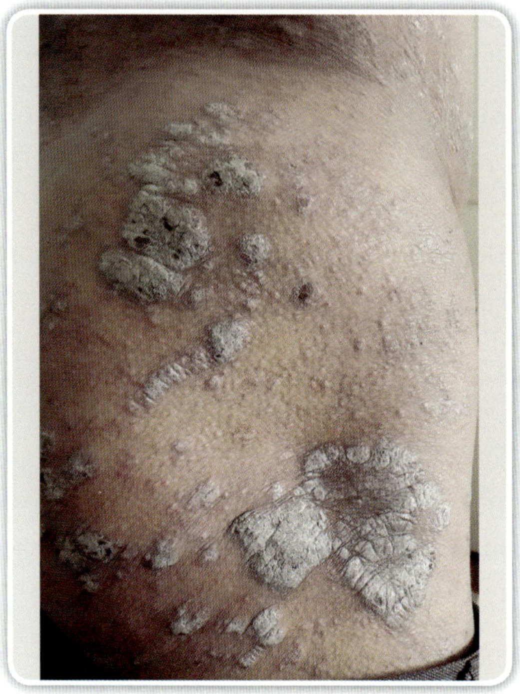

FIG. 8.68: Multiple plaques of rupioid psoriasis over the back in same patient

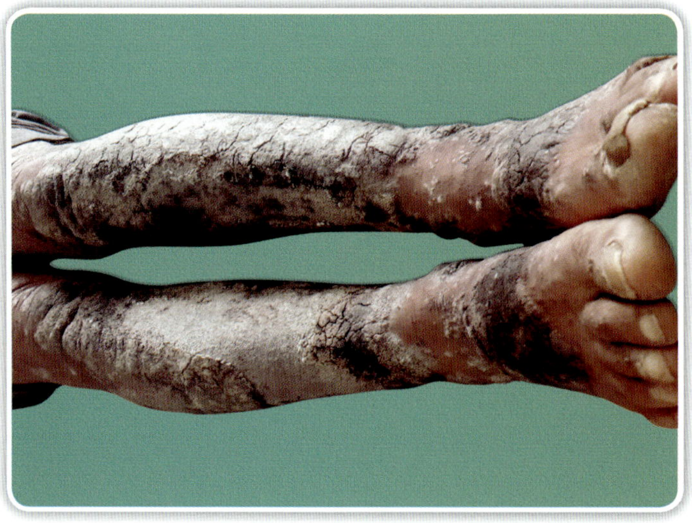

FIG. 8.69: Same patient showing rupioid psoriatic plaques involving both the lower limbs

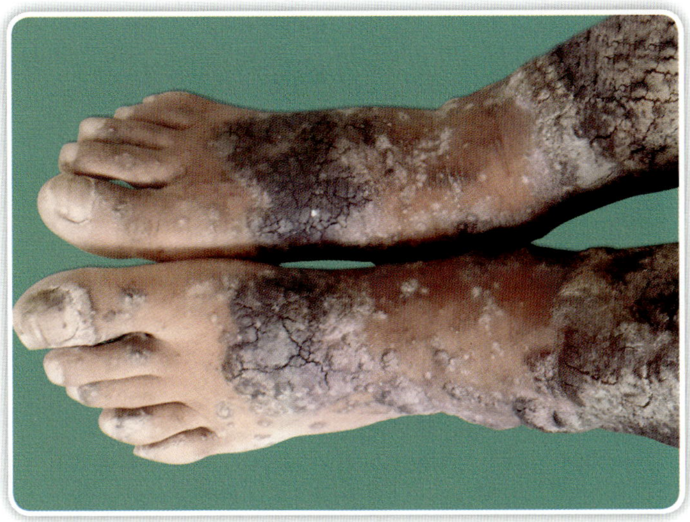

FIG. 8.70: A closer view of rupioid psoriatic plaques involving feet and digits in same patient

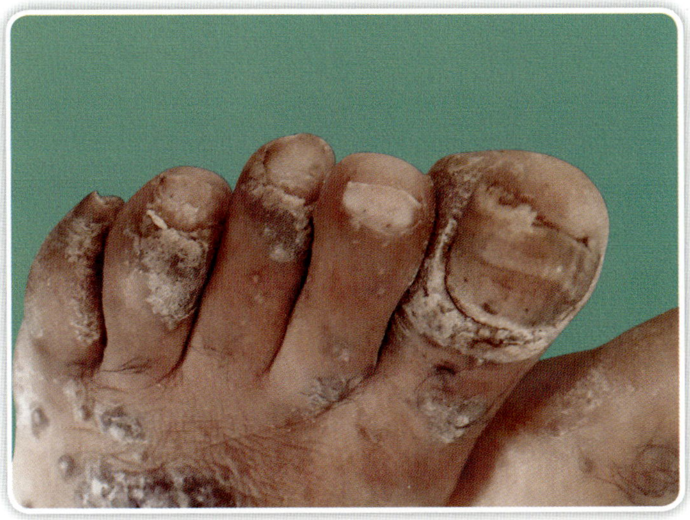

FIG. 8.71: Nail and periungual involvement in the same patient with rupioid psoriasis

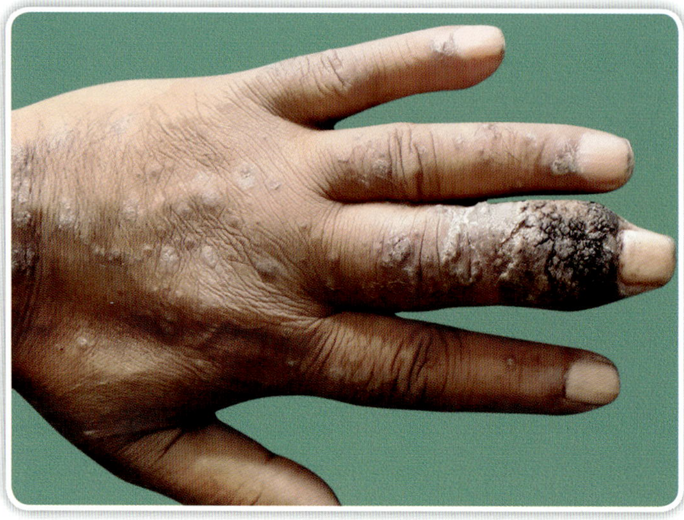

FIG. 8.72: Rupioid psoriatic plaque involving the left middle finger

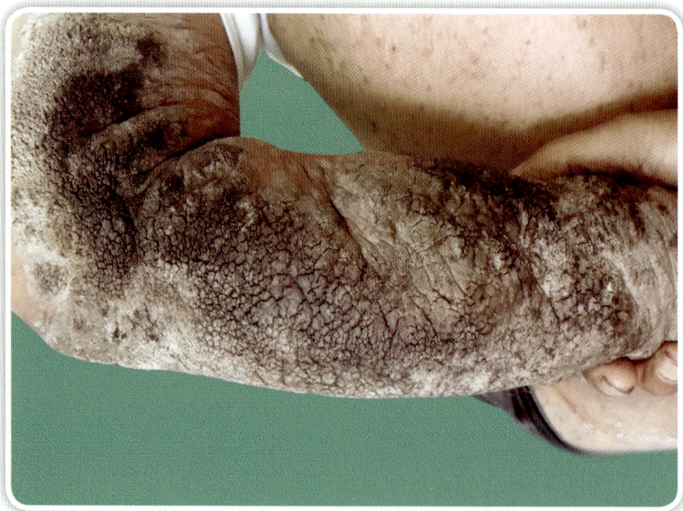

FIG. 8.73: Rupioid psoriatic plaques involving the right arm and forearm

Linear Naevoid Psoriasis

It is characterised by a linear distribution of psoriatic lesions along Blaschko's lines. True linear psoriasis in the absence of lesions elsewhere is rare with only few cases reported in the literature. Happle has proposed the pathogenesis of linear psoriasis as somatic recombination of a gene predisposing to psoriasis leading to segmental mosaicism (Fig. 8.74).[25]

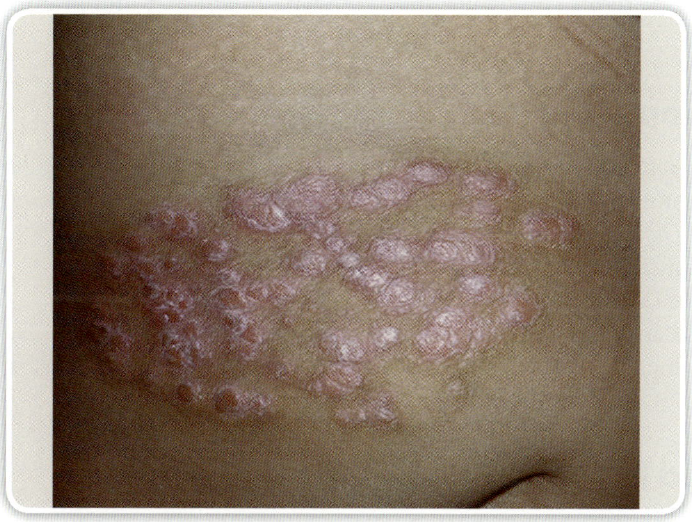

FIG. 8.74: Picture showing segmental distribution of psoriatic lesions on the abdomen in an 8 year old girl. She had similar lesions on the ipsilateral side of neck

Unstable Psoriasis

This term is used to describe the phases of disease in which activity is marked and the course and immediate outcome is unpredictable; for example, in stages when a previously stable and chronic form is exacerbated by inappropriate management and threatens to become erythrodermic or pustular, or when localized pustular or ill-defined erythematous lesions appear spontaneously for the first time. Patients may develop such unstable phases repeatedly settling back again into the classical forms of the disease. Withdrawal of intensive systemic or topical corticosteroid therapy, hypocalcemia, acute infection, overtreatment with tar, dithranol or UV-irradiation and perhaps severe emotional upset may precipitate this condition.[26]

PUSTULAR PSORIASIS

Pustular psoriasis is an uncommon form of psoriasis consisting of widespread pustules on an erythematous background. In pustular psoriasis, pus-filled lesions called pustules develop on skin over an erythematous (red) background. Although pustules are typically associated with infection, in pustular psoriasis the lesions are formed as the result of inflammation, usually in the absence of infection. Both generalized and localized types of pustular psoriasis are recognized.[27]

Clinical Features

There are multiple variants of pustular psoriasis; they can be subdivided into generalized and localized variants. Patients can evolve from one type to another and manifest other forms of psoriasis as well.

Classification

A convenient classification is as follows.

1. Localised pustular psoriasis: Includes palmoplantar pustulosis and acrodermatitis continua.
2. Generalised pustular psoriasis (GPP): Includes acute **(Von Zumbusch)**, GPP of pregnancy, infantile and juvenile, circinate and localized (not hands and feet) types.

Generalized Forms

Von Zumbusch pustular psoriasis is the prototype of generalized pustular psoriasis and can be life-threatening but is rare. It is characterized by a sudden appearance of sheets of sterile white-yellow pustules over an erythematous background. The pustules coalesce into larger lakes of pus and the skin can be quite tender to touch. There may be involvement of mucous membranes (which is rarely seen in stable forms of psoriasis), in the form of a fissured and erythematous tongue. The acute onset, often within hours, is accompanied by fever, headache and malaise and it can persist for weeks if not treated. Hospital admission is usually required and pustules resolve over several days to weeks, leaving large areas of scaling behind (Figs 8.75 to 8.86).[28]

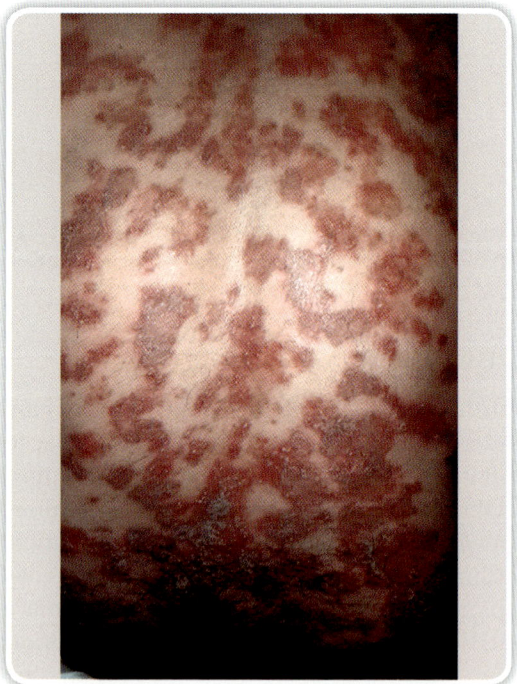

FIG. 8.75: Generalised pustular psoriasis with pustules at the periphery of psoriatic plaques in a patient

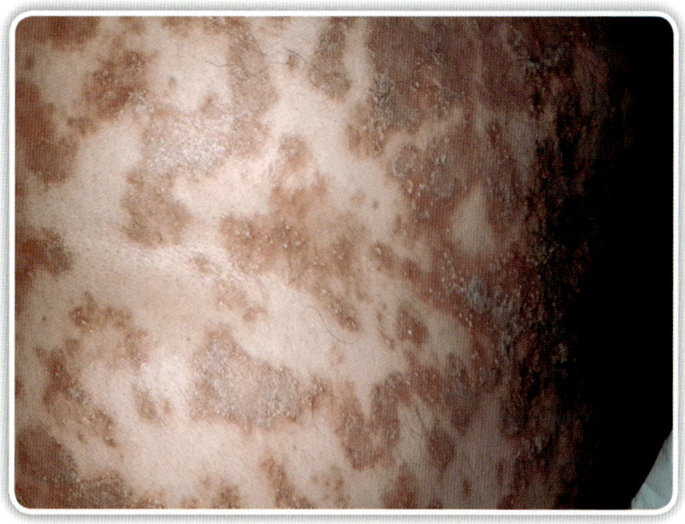

FIG. 8.76: Same patient with lakes of pus

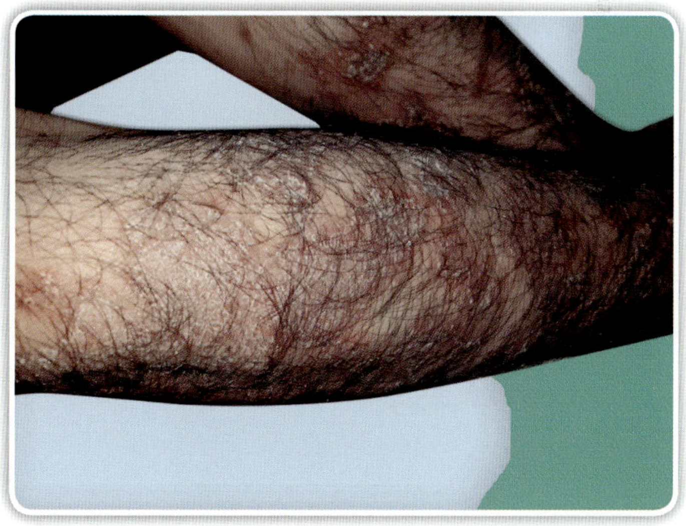

FIG. 8.77: Same patient showing pustular psoriatic plaques involving the limbs

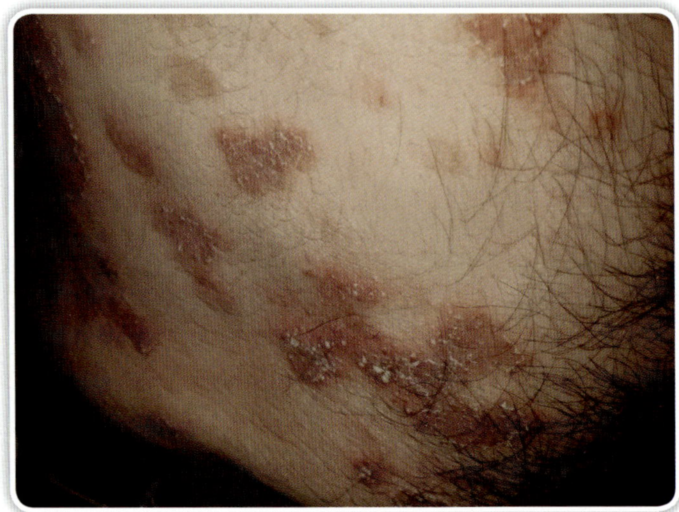

FIG. 8.78: Another patient with generalized pustular psoriasis showing multiple sterile pustules

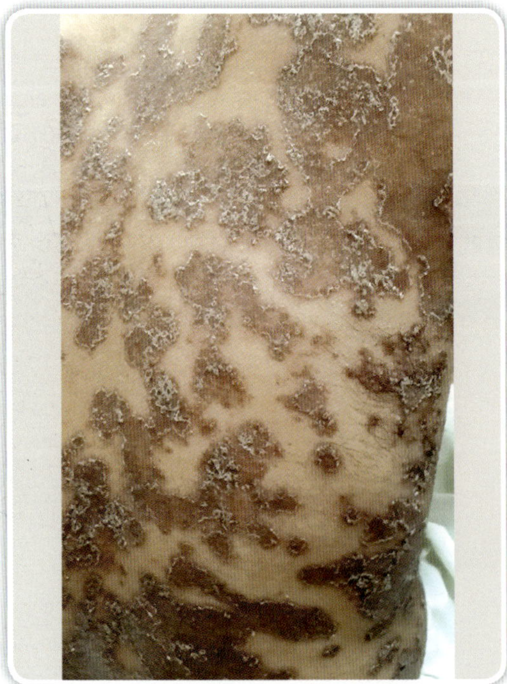

FIG. 8.79: Generalized pustular psoriasis in a young boy with Down's syndrome

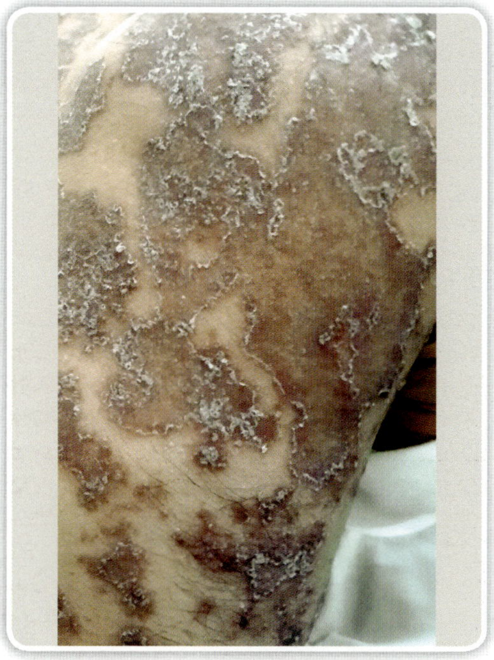

FIG. 8.80: Same patient showing desquamating lesions with active lesions of pustular psoriasis

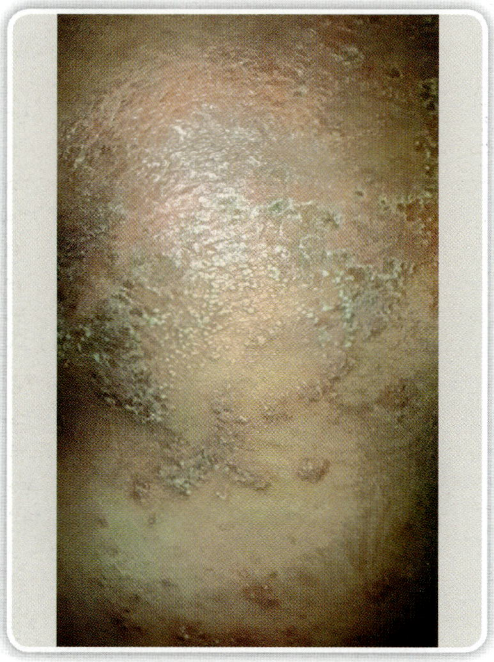

FIG. 8.81: Same patient showing multiple pinpoint pustules overlying psoriatic plaques

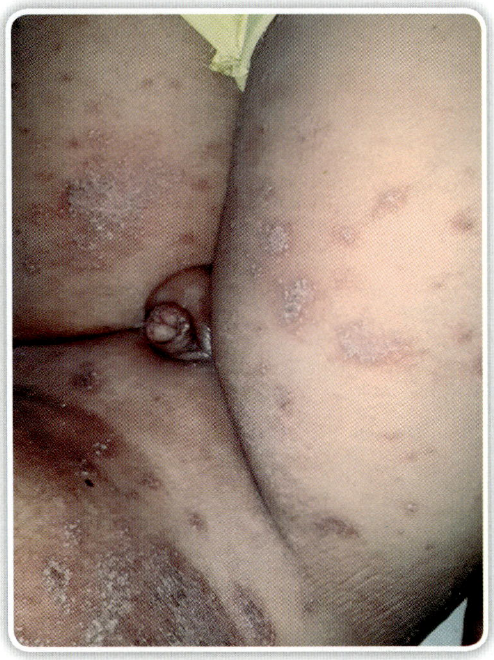

FIG. 8.82: Same patient showing pustular lesions over the abdomen, thighs and genital region

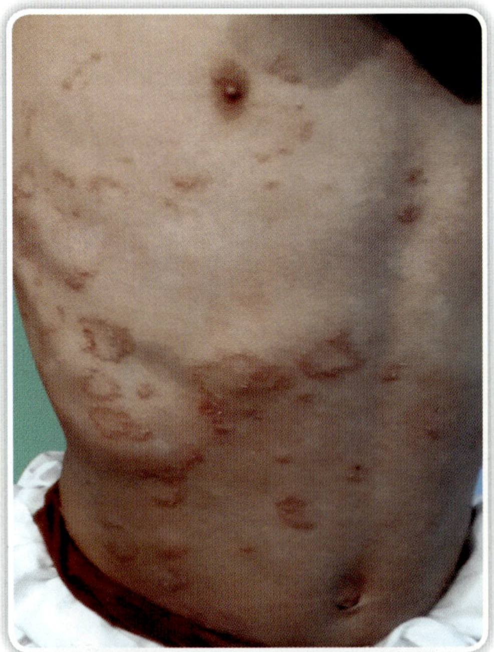

FIG. 8.83: Another patient of generalized pustular psoriasis with peripheral pustules and central clearing of plaques

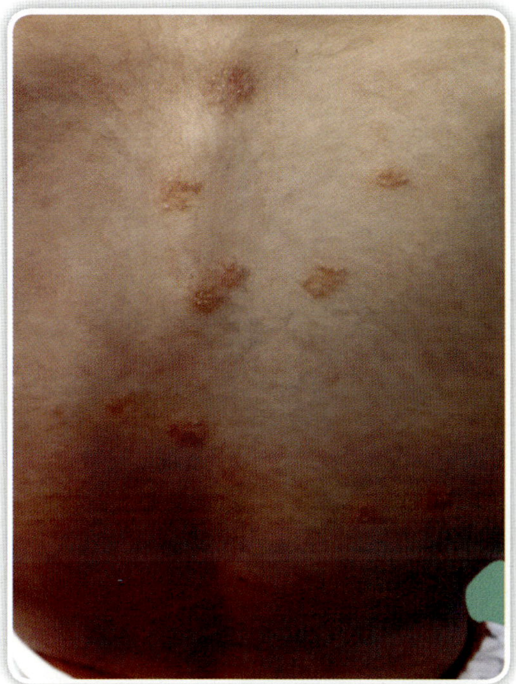

FIG. 8.84: Same patient with pustular psoriatic lesions over the back

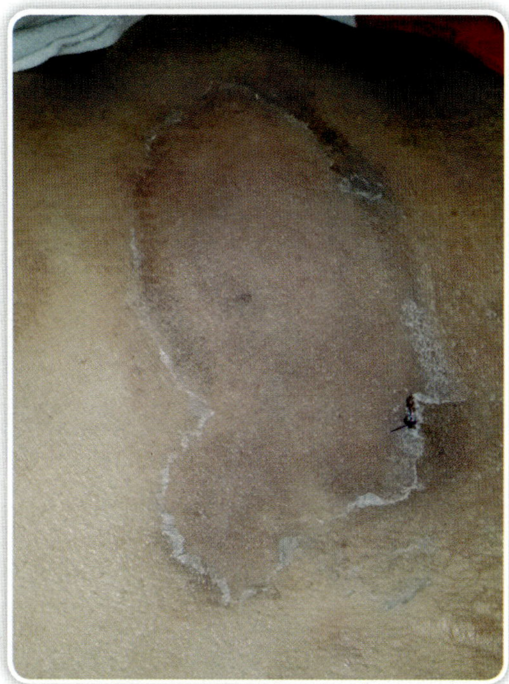

FIG. 8.85: Resolving pustular psoriatic plaque over the back in a female patient

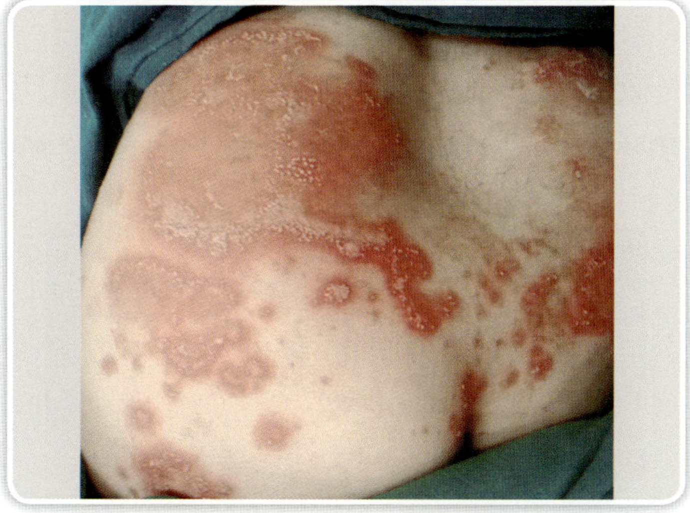

FIG. 8.86: Picture showing generalized pustular psoriasis with sterile pustules at the periphery of psoriatic plaques.

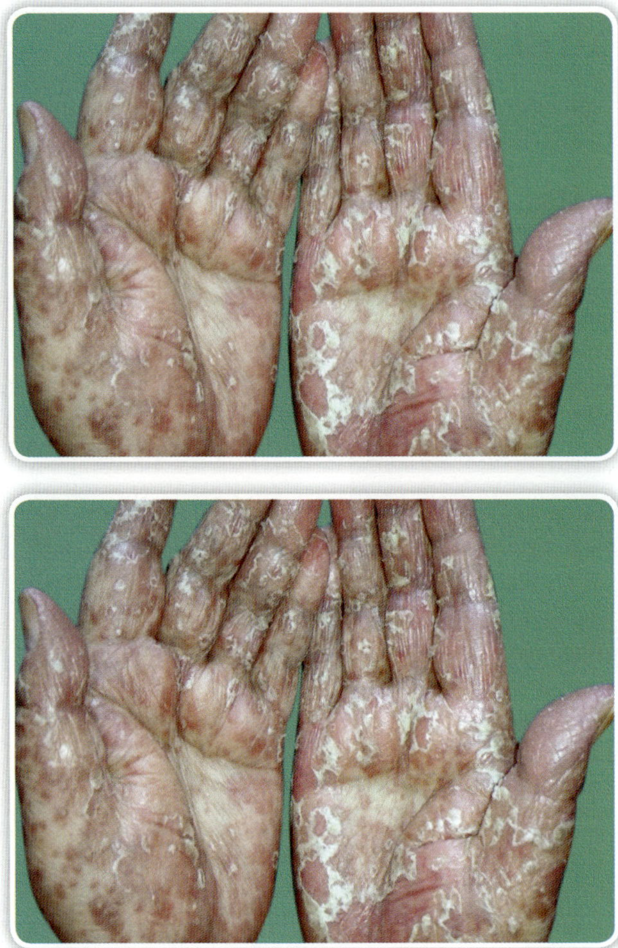

FIG. 8.87: Pustular psoriatic lesions involving the palms. Note the deep-red erythema

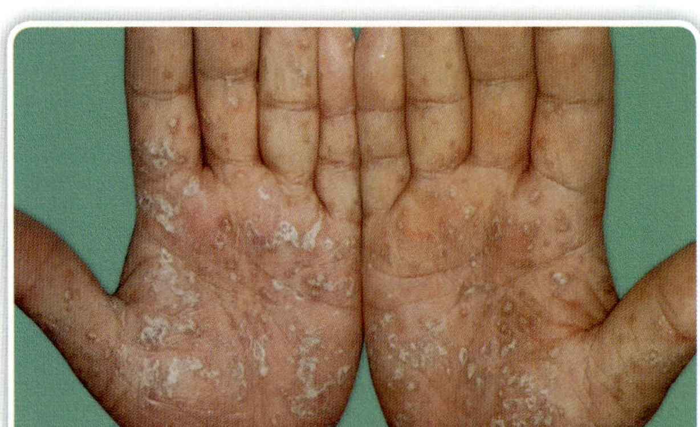

FIG. 8.88: Another patient showing pustular psoriatic lesions involving the palms

Impetigo herpetiformis is a variant of pustular psoriasis that occurs during pregnancy. Otherwise, it is similar to the von Zumbusch variety. Generalized pustules with fever and leukocytosis is seen.[29]

Annular GPP is a variant of psutular psoriasis which is more commonly seen in infants and it manifests with annular lesions surrounded by pustules. As the lesions grow, the center clears with desquamation. At times, associated symptoms such as fever, malaise and local tenderness may be associated.

In the **exanthematic type**, there are no systemic symptoms. Patients present with an acute eruption of small pustules, which last several days, then clearing completely. It tends to follow infections or drug-intake. There may be some overlap with a pustular drug eruption called acute generalized exanthematous pustulosis (AGEP).

Infantile and juvenile type: It is very rare with course being benign and characterized by spontaneous remissions and onset usually in the first few weeks of life. A history of napkin dermatitis, sudden-onset napkin psoriasis or seborrhoeic dermatitis may be obtained.

Circinate, annular and linear pustular psoriasis: These are seen usually in subacute or chronic forms of the widespread pustular psoriasis. The lesions begin as discrete areas of erythema, which become raised and edematous. Slow centrifugal spread usually occurs. Pustules appear peripherally on the crest of the advancing edge, become desiccated and leave behind a trailing fringe of scale as the lesion slowly advances.[30,31]

Localized Forms

Palmoplantar pustulosis is a chronic variant that occurs mainly in women, usually in their 5th and 6th decades. Triggers include smoking, stress and infections. Pustules with yellow-brown macules on the palms and soles and scaly red plaques are usually present. The condition can be associated with bony lesions (e.g. SAPHO syndrome—synovitis, acne, pustulosis, hyperostosis, osteitis).

Acrodermatitis continua of Hallopeau is a rare form of psoriasis affecting digits and nails. Pustules form on the fingers and toes, progressing to crusts with scale formation. There is loss of the nail if the nail bed is affected (Figs 8.77 and 8.88).[32,33]

Risk Factors

The following factors can reportedly trigger an eruption of pustular psoriasis:

- Withdrawal of systemic steroids
- Drugs, including salicylates, iodine, lithium, phenylbutazone, oxyphenbutazone, trazodone, penicillin, hydroxychloroquine, calcipotriol, interferon-alpha and recombinant interferon-beta
- Strong irritating topicals, including tar, anthralin, steroids under occlusion and zinc pyrithione in shampoo
- Infections
- Sunlight or phototherapy
- Cholestatic jaundice
- Hypocalcemia
- Idiopathic.[34,35]

Management Including Investigations and Diagnosis[36,37]

The differential diagnosis includes other dermatoses that manifest with pustules, including drug reactions, infections and bullous diseases. A complete blood count often shows leukocytosis and an elevated erythrocyte sedimentation rate. Consider a serum calcium profile, renal function and liver function tests, prior to starting systemic medication. Swabbing a pustule for culture and sensitivity is indicated if an infectious cause is suspected, e.g. folliculitis, impetigo. All patients with psoriasis should be screened for psoriatic arthritis. Imaging and a rheumatology referral should be considered as needed.

Immediate Care

Generalized flares of pustular psoriasis are life-threatening and often mandate hospital admission. There is a risk of high-output cardiac failure, hypocalcemia, hypoalbuminemia, renal failure and bacterial superinfection.

Treatment

In addition to supportive care, a number of treatment options are available for pustular psoriasis. Topical corticosteroids can work well for limited variants, but systemic corticosteroids are reserved for special cases such as impetigo herpetiformis, where they are the safest aggressive option during pregnancy. After delivery, patients can be switched to more potent therapies, such as systemic retinoids or steroid-sparing agents, e.g. methotrexate.

Systemic retinoids are often very effective and are considered first-line therapy for GPP. Oral acitretin can be quite fast-acting, but isotretinoin is preferred for women of child-bearing age because it has a shorter period of teratogenicity. Other systemic options with demonstrated efficacy include methotrexate, usually started at 15 mg weekly and cyclosporine at 4–5 mg/kg daily. Biologics, e.g. TNF-alpha inhibitors, may also be considered.

If the above mentioned treatments do not work then alternative therapies, such as colchicine at 0.6 mg PO 2–3 times/day as tolerated, mycophenolate mofetil, azathioprine, or hydroxyurea can be tried.

Points to Remember

- Plaque psoriasis is the most common type of psoriasis
- Systemic retinoids are the treatment of first choice for GPP
- Systemic steroids are usually contraindicated in psoriasis except for the treatment of impetigo herpetiformis

REFERENCE

1. Lowes MA, Bowcock AM, Krueger JG. Pathogenesis and therapy of psoriasis. Nature. 2007;22(445):866-73.
2. Griffiths CE, Barker JN. Pathogenesis and clinical features of psoriasis. Lancet. 2007;21(370):263-71.
3. Camisa C. Psoriasis. Boston: Blackwell; 1994. pp. 32-3.
4. Whyte HJ, Baughmann RD. Acute guttate psoriasis and streptococcal infection. Arch Dermatol. 1964;89:350.

5. Braverman JM, Cohen I, O'Keefe E. Metabolic and ultrastructural studies in a patient with pustular psoriasis. Arch Dermatol. 1972;105:189.
6. Everall J. Intractable pustular eruptions of the hands and feet. Br J Dermatol. 1957;69:269-72.
7. Rym BM, Mourad M, Bechir Z, et al. Erythroderma in adults: A report of 80 cases. Int J Dermatol. 2005;44(9):731-5.
8. Rosenbach M, Hsu S, Korman NJ, et al. Treatment of erythrodermic psoriasis: From the medical board of the National Psoriasis Foundation. J Am Acad Dermatol. 2010;62(4):655-62.
9. Ahdout J, Mandel H, Chiu M. Erythroderma in a patient taking acitretin for plaque psoriasis. J Drugs Dermatol. 2008;7(4):391-4.
10. Marks J. Erythroderma and its management. Clin Exp Dermatol. 1982;7:415-22.
11. Shuster S. Psoriatic alopecia. Br J Dermatol. 1972;87:73-7.
12. William J, Timothy B, Dirk E. Andrews' Diseases of the Skin: Clinical Dermatology, (10th ed). Saunders; 2005. ISBN 0-7216-2921-0.
13. Kouskoukis C, Scher R, Ackerman A. "The "oil drop" sign of psoriatic nails. A clinical finding specific for psoriasis". The Am J Dermatopathol. 1983;5(3):259-62.
14. Kaur I, Kumar B, Sharma VK, Kaur S. Epidemiology of psoriasis in a clinic from North India. Indian J Dermatol Venereol Leprol. 1986;52:208-12.
15. Ghosal A,Gangopadhyay DN,Chanda M,Das NK.Sudy of nail changes in psoriasis.Indian J Dermatol 2004;49:18-21.
16. Rich P, Scher R. "Nail Psoriasis Severity Index: A useful tool for evaluation of nail psoriasis". J Am Acad Dermatol. 2003;49(2):206-12.
17. Zaias N. Psoriasis of the nail. Arch Dermatol. 1969;99:567-79.
18. Parrish CA, Sobera JO, Elewski BE. "Modification of the Nail Psoriasis Severity Index." J Am Acad Dermatol. 2005;53(4):745-6.
19. Rigopoulos D, Gregoriou S, Daniel III CR, Belyayeva H, Larios G, Verra P, et al. "Treatment of Nail Psoriasis with a Two-Compound Formulation of Calcipotriol plus Betamethasone Dipropionate Ointment". Dermatology. 2009;218(4):338-41.
20. Saleem K, Azim W. "Treatment of nail psoriasis with a modified regimen of steroid injections". J Coll Physicians Surg Pak. 2008;18(2):78-81.
21. Zaias N, editor. The nail in health and disease. Lancaster. UK: MTP Press Ltd; 1980.
22. Tosti A, Fanti PA, Morelli R, Bardazzi F. Psoriasiform acral dermatitis. Acta Derm Venereol. 1992;72:206-7.
23. Birnbaum RY, Zvulunov A, Hallel-Halevy D, et al. Seborrhoea like dermatitis with psoriasiform elements caused by a mutation in ZNF750, encoding a putative C2H2 zinc finger motif. Nature Genet. 2006;38:749-51.
24. Stevanovich DV. Rarities in the clinical picture of psoriasis. Acta Derma Venereol. 1979;59(87):98.
25. Kerl H, Pachinger W. Psoriasis:odd varieties in the adult. Acta Derma Venereol. 1979;59(87):90-4.
26. Ingram JT. The significance and management of psoriasis. BMJ. 1954;II:823-8.
27. Baker H, Ryan TJ. Generalised pustular psoriasis. Br J Dermatol. 1986;80:771-93.
28. Von Zumbusch LR. Psoriasis and pustuloses Exanthem. Arch Dermatol Syphilol. 1910;99:335-46.
29. Feiwel M, Ferriman D. Impetigo herpetiformis. Proc R Soc Med. 1957;50:392-4.
30. Baker H. Pustular psoriasis. Dermatol Clin. 1984;2:455-70.
31. Degos R, Civatte J, Arrouy M. Psoriasis et psoriasis pustuleux a type d'erytheme annulaire centrifuge (3 cas). Bull Soc Fr Dermatol Syphiligr. 1966;73:356-8.
32. Reitamo S, Erkko P, Remitz A. Palmoplantar pustulosis. Eur J Dermatol. 1992;2:311-4.
33. Thomsen K, Osterbye P. Pustulosis Palmaris et plantaris. Br J Dermatol. 1973;89:293-6.
34. Baker H. Corticosteroids and pustular psoriasis. Br J Dermatol. 1976;94(12):83-8.
35. Shelly WB. Generalised pustular psoriasis induced by potassium iodide. JAMA. 1967;201:1009-14.
36. Ozawa A, Ohkido M, Haraki Y. Treatment of generalised pustular psoriasis: A multicentre study in Japan. J Dermatol. 1999;26:141-9.
37. Piamphongsant T, Nimsuwan P, Gritiyarangsan P. Treatment of generalised pustular psoriasis: Clinical trials using different therapeutic modalities. Clin Exp Dermatol. 1985;10:552-61.

Chapter

9

Assessing the Severity of Psoriasis

While all types of psoriasis are well defined, parameters to describe the severity of psoriasis have not yet been clearly laid out. Perhaps the largest drawback is that the description of severe psoriasis varies depending upon the judgment of the assessor. One patient may define it differently from another depending upon how it is affecting his or her quality of life. There are also a number of different techniques used to measure the severity of psoriasis. Furthermore, clinicians need to establish whether the severity is comparative or absolute, or current or long term.

Psoriasis area severity index (PASI) *is widely used in clincial trials.*

Psoriasis area and severity index is the most widely used tool for the measurement of severity of psoriasis. PASI combines the assessment of the severity of lesions and the area affected into a single score in the range 0 (no disease) to 72 (maximal disease).

The body is divided into four sections (head (H) (10% of a person's skin); arms (A) (20%); trunk (T) (30%); legs (L) (40%)). Each of these areas is scored by itself and then the four scores are combined into the final PASI. For each section, the percent of area of skin involved, is estimated and then transformed into a grade from 0 to 6:

- 0% of involved area—grade 0
- <10% of involved area—grade 1
- 10–29% of involved area—grade 2
- 30–49% of involved area—grade 3
- 50–69% of involved area—grade 4
- 70–89% of involved area—grade 5
- 90–100% of involved area—grade 6

Within each area, the severity is estimated by three clinical signs: Erythema (redness), induration (thickness) and desquamation (scaling). Severity parameters are measured on a scale of 0–4, from none to maximum.

The sum of all three severity parameters is then calculated for each section of skin, multiplied by the area score for that area and multiplied by weight of respective section (0.1 for head, 0.2 for arms, 0.3 for trunk and 0.4 for legs).

The **adapted PASI index,** where the psoriatic area is not converted into an area grade, but is maintained as a continuous variable, improves the power of the clinical trial. The modified PASI which involves computer-aided area measurement as a continuous variable is named computer-aided psoriasis continuous area and severity score cPcASI.

One common method for measuring psoriasis severity is based on the percentage of affected body surface. For example, one palm-sized lesion represents 1% of body surface area (BSA).

- Mild psoriasis affects <3% of BSA
- Moderate psoriasis affects 3–10% of BSA
- Severe psoriasis affects >10% of BSA.

SALFORD PSORIASIS INDEX

Salford psoriasis index (SPI) is a new scoring system for psoriasis. It incorporates the current clinical extent of psoriasis based on the psoriasis area and severity index (PASI), which is transformed into a score from 0 to 10, a score indicating psychosocial disability (0–10 on visual analogue scale) and past severity based on treatment history (which reflects the historical severity of disease as judged by the need for systemic treatment, admission to hospital and number of episodes of erythroderma).

The measure of social, emotional and fuctional impairment resulting from psoriasis is critical. The **Dermatology life quality index (DLQI)** questionnaire is a commonly used tool to assess patient reported outcomes. In one study about 48% of psoriasis patients reported adverse impacts on social functioning, leading to decreased work efficiency in 51% and to workplace distress in 63%. Stress in the home environment and interpersonal relationships were reported by 70%.[1,2]

Techniques used to measure the severity of psoriasis

- Body surface area
- Dermatology life quality index (DLQI)
- Lattice system physician's global assessment (LS-PGA)
- National psoriasis foundation psoriasis score (NPF-PS)
- Physician's global assessment
- Psoriasis area and severity index
- Psoriasis symptom assessment
- Salford psoriasis index
- Self-administered PASI (SAPASI)

REFERENCES

1. Langley RG, Ellis CN. Evaluating psoriasis with Psoriasis Area and Severity Index, Psoriasis Global Assessment, and Lattice System Physician's Global Assessment. J Am Acad Dermatol. 2004;51:563-9.
2. Carlin CS, Feldman SR, Krueger JG, Menter A, Krueger GG. A 50% reduction in the Psoriasis Area and Severity Score (PASI 50) is a clinically significant endpoint in the assessment of psoriasis. J Am Acad Dermatol. 2004;50:859-66.

Chapter

10

History of the Disease and Triggers

The current evidence indicates that the interaction between genes and the environment are important in disease association. Many environmental factors have been linked to psoriasis and have been implicated in the initiation and exacerbation of psoriasis. Following are the factors which are implicated in the initiation and exacerbation of psoriasis.

1. *Trauma:* Physical, chemical, electrical, surgical, infective and inflammatory stimuli have been reported to elicit psoriatic lesions (Koebner phenomenon).[1]
2. *Infections:* A strong association between pharyngitis by group A beta-hemolytic streptococci and the clinical activity of psoriasis (guttate psoriasis) is now well established and accounts for the clinical efficacy of penicillins and rifampicin.[2]
3. *Drugs:* There are a number of drugs which have been reported to be responsible for the onset or exacerbation of psoriasis.[3]

   Drugs that precipitate or exacerbate psoriasis.

   - Angiotensin-converting enzyme (ACE) inhibitors
   - Beta-blockers
   - Interferons
   - Lithium
   - Non-steroidal anti-inflammatory drugs (NSAIDS)
   - Tetracyclines

   Drug-provoked psoriasis has been divided into two types viz; Drug induced and drug aggravated types. The drug-induced psoriasis is where discontinuation of the causative drug stops the further progression of the disease and the drug-aggravated psoriasis, is where the disease progresses even after the discontinuation of the offending drug. True drug-induced psoriasis has been noted to occur in a de-novo fashion in patients with no family or previous history of psoriasis. The clinical presentation of these lesions may often mimic the pustular variant of psoriasis, often with no nail involvement or associated arthritis. Furthermore, there is an absence of Munro microabscesses, few macrophages and sparse vascular changes noted histologically. In contrast the drug-aggravated psoriasis exhibits a propensity to occur in patients with a history of psoriasis or with a genetic predisposition for the disease. Patients can have exacerbation of preexisting psoriatic lesions or develop new lesions in previously uninvolved skin. Histological examination reveals features that are more characteristic of psoriasis vulgaris.

   Mechanism of induction/aggravation of psoriasis by beta-blockers.

   Various theories that have been proposed regarding the pathogenesis of beta-blocker induced psoriasis are as follows:

1. Immunological mechanisms including impaired lymphocyte transformation and a delayed type hypersensitivity reaction.
2. Alterations in the cyclic adenosine monophosphate (cAMP) pathway. Cyclic adenosine monophosphate is an intracellular messenger that is responsible for the stimulation of proteins for cellular differentiation and inhibition of proliferation. It has been suggested that the blockade of epidermal β_2 receptors leads to a decrease in intraepidermal cAMP causing keratinocyte hyperproliferation. Both cardioselective as well as nonselective groups of beta-blockers exhibit excessive release of enzymes by lymphocytes, neutrophils and macrophages and it is believed that this event is responsible for the presence of hyperproliferation and psoriasiform change.
3. Beta-blockers have been reported to increase phosphorylation in T cells in psoriasis, which may be relevant to intracellular levels of calcium. The blockade of these receptors has been implicated in the pathogenesis of drug-provoked psoriasis in both groups of beta-blockers.

Mechanism of induction/aggravation of psoriasis by lithium

The proposed hypotheses for the induction/aggravation of psoriasis by lithium are as follows:

1. Lithium causes depletion of inositol monophosphatase resulting in alterations in calcium homeostasis and seritonergic function. Inositol monophosphate is an intracellular second messenger system linked to neurotransmitters affecting cell function, growth and differentiation. The association between the blockade of the phosphatidyl inositol pathway and lithium-provoked psoriasis is through the release and depletion of intracellular calcium. Low intracellular calcium levels cause increased proliferation of keratinocytes and affect terminal differentiation.
2. Lithium treatment has been shown to decrease cAMP levels, which in turn decreases the intracellular levels of calcium, hence leading to a lack of differentiation, increased proliferation of keratinocytes and enhanced chemotaxis and phagocytic activity of polymorphonuclear leukocytes.
3. Lithium has been reported to increase the intracellular tyrosine phosphorylation in psoriatic T cells but not in control T cells, with a possible implication to psoriasis development.

4. *Sunlight:* Sunlight is generally beneficial in psoriasis, although summer exacerbations are well known. Photosensitive psoriasis is seen predominantly in females, is strongly associated with females and HLA-cw6 and is seen in early-onset psoriasis.[4]
5. *Metabolic factors:* Psoriatic patients have an increased risk of developing metabolic syndrome, including obesity, diabetes, hyperlipidemia and hypertension.The early onset of psoriasis in women, with a peak around puberty, changes during pregnany (improves more than worsens) and provocation of psoriasis by high-dose estrogen therapy potentially indicates a role for hormonal factors in the disease. Hypocalcemia has been reported to occur in severe forms of the disease particularly generalized pustular psoriasis and may be a predictor of poor outcome.[5]
6. *Psychogenic factors:* Psoriasis produces significant adverse effects on the psychological and social aspects of life mainly because of its visibility. There are few studies from India addressing this aspect of the disease. Psoriasis sufferers feel self-conscious, disturbed/inconvenienced by the shedding of the skin, live in a constant fear of relapse and avoid social interactions.[6]

7. *Alcohol and smoking:* Both alcohol and smoking have been reported to have a detrimental effect on psoriasis, although the exact association is not known.These two factors are more common in males than females and abstinence has been reported to induce remission.[7]
8. *HIV and acquired immune deficiency syndrome:* Severe psoriasis and psoriatic arthropathy has been reported in patients with HIV. The prognosis of AIDS is also poor in patients with severe psoriasis.[8]

The goal of control versus cure is a more practical outcome of treatment. Many randomized controlled clinical trials involving children under the age of 12 years have reported on two topical treatments: Calcipotriol and corticosteroids. Avoidance of triggers like trauma (Koebner phenomenon), including physical, surgical, or inflammatory trauma, should be borne in mind in this age group. A strong association between pharyngitis by group A beta-hemolytic streptococci and the clinical activity of psoriasis (guttate psoriasis) is now well established and should be properly investigated where relevant.

REFERENCES

1. Eyre RW, Krueger GG. The Koebner response in psoriasis. In:Roenigk HH, Maibach HI, eds. Psoriasis. New York: Marcel Dekker; 1984. pp. 1:05-16.
2. Telfer NR, Chalmers RJ, Whale K, Colman G. The role of streptococcal infection in the initiation of guttate psoriasis. Arch Dermatol. 1992;128:39-42.
3. Abel EA, DiCicco LM, Orenberg EK, et al. Drugs in exacerbation of psoriasis. J Am Acad Dermatol. 1986;15: 1007-22.
4. Ros AM, Eklund G. Photosensitive psoriasis. J Am Acad Dermatol. 1987;17:752-8.
5. Dunna SF, Finlay AY. Psoriasis: Improvement during and worsening after pregnancy. Br J Dermatol. 1996;120:584.
6. Seville RH. Psoriasis and stress. Br J Dermatol. 1977;97:279-302.
7. Higgins E. Alcohol, smoking and psoriasis. Clin Exp Dermatol. 2000;25:107-10.
8. Johnson TM, Duvic M, Rapini RP, et al. Acquired immune deficiency syndrome (AIDS) can exacerbate psoriasis. J Am Acad Dermatol. 1988;88:144.

Chapter

11 Effects of Psoriasis

Psoriasis among all the cutaneous diseases probably, is associated with high morbidity and a great level of psychological stress due to visible disability. Females tend to be affected more than males. Socially and economically, patients with psoriasis tend to have a lower income, reduced levels of employment and a poorer quality of life, due to isolation and depression associated with the disease. The National Psoriasis Foundation found a moderate to large negative impact of the disease on the quality of life of patients, with an alteration of everyday activities. Impaired health-related quality of life may lead to unhealthy lifestyle behaviors, such as smoking, alcohol consumption, decreased physical activity and obesity, which are independent risk factors for cardiovascular diseases. In contrast, it is possible that obesity favors psoriasis in predisposed individuals because of the proinflammatory state and release of inflammatory mediators, such as adipocytokines. Various studies have shown that, the greater the body surface area involvement, the lower the quality of life. Depressive illness in psoriasis is associated with a low self esteem, a fear of public rejection and psychosexual concerns. Although not much research has been conducted in this area, it has been shown that psoriasis also impacts the quality of life of family members and partners. The various effects of psoriasis on different body systems are summarised below.

PHYSICAL

Various studies have shown that psoriasis is associated with a range of medical comorbidities including coronary artery disease, metabolic syndrome, renal failure, liver disease, viral hepatitis B or C, asthma, peptic ulcers and malignancies, whereby the extent of the comorbidity increases with the severity of the psoriasis. One study group has postulated that there might be a genetic link between psoriasis and these comorbidities. There also seems to be a relationship between inflammatory factors in psoriasis and those with streptococcal oropharyngeal infections, decreased responsiveness to allergens and a decreased frequency of rheumatic fever and poststreptococcal nephritis.[1]

PSORIATIC ARTHRITIS

Psoriatic arthritis is a seronegative inflammatory arthritis that occurs in the presence of skin or nail psoriasis. It can be divided into five types: Distal interphalangeal joint, asymmetrical oligoarthritis, polyarthritis, spondylitis and arthritis mutilans. It resembles rheumatoid arthritis in its effects. This complication of psoriasis can cause joint damage and a loss of function in some joints, which can be debilitating.[2]

CARDIOVASCULAR DISEASE AND METABOLIC SYNDROME

The risk of cardiovascular disease in psoriatic patients increases by threefold with moderate and severe disease, but there is no apparent risk in those with mild disease. It is thought that the chronic systemic inflammation associated with psoriasis results in coronary artery disease (CAD), because the inflammatory mediators of psoriasis are similar to those of CAD. Psoriatic patients also have an increased risk of developing metabolic syndrome, including obesity, diabetes, hyperlipidemia and hypertension.[3]

CROHN'S DISEASE

Crohn's disease is seen seven times more often in psoriatic patients. This may be due to overlapping inflammatory pathways common in both conditions or be a side effect of some of the biological agents used in the management of psoriasis, such as infliximab and adalimumab.[4]

MALIGNANCIES

Some authors postulate that psoriasis may be associated with an increased risk of nonmelanoma skin cancers; however, this could be a side effect of psoriasis treatments, including photochemotherapy.[5]

Ocular effects: Certain eye disorders, such as conjunctivitis, blepharitis and uveitis are more common in people with psoriasis.

Obesity: People with psoriasis, especially those with more severe disease, are more likely to be obese. It is not clear how these two diseases are linked, however. It has been suggested that obesity favors psoriasis in predisposed individuals because of the proinflammatory state and release of inflammatory mediators, such as adipocytokines. People with psoriasis are also more likely to gain weight due to sedentary lifestyle (possibly due to isolation and social rejection).[6]

Type 2 diabetes: The risk of type 2 diabetes is increased in people with psoriasis, possibly due to increased incidence of metabolic syndrome in them. It has been suggested that the risk of acquiring type 2 diabetes increases with increasing severity of the disease.

High blood pressure: Various studies have shown increased prevalence of hypertension in people with psoriasis, possibly due to increased association of metabolic syndrome and CAD.

Other autoimmune diseases: Celiac disease, systemic sclerosis and Crohn's disease have been shown to affect people with psoriasis more often. In some studies the incidence of these diseases is more than five times in patients with psoriasis.[7]

Parkinson's disease: This chronic neurological condition with significant morbidity and impact on the quality of life of patient and his or her family members, has been reported to occur in people with psoriasis more than the control population.

Psoriasis can also affect the quality of life by increasing the risk of the following:

- Low self-esteem
- Depression
- Social isolation
- Problems at work, which can lead to a lower income.

It is the proper and timely management and counselling that can decrease the impact of psoriasis on various body systems and hence improve the quality of life.

Points to Remember

- Psoriasis is associated with a high morbidity and a great level of psychological stress (depression is more common)
- Metabolic syndrome, autoimmune diseases, Parkinson's disease, hypertension, obesity, Type 2 diabetes and psoriatic arthritis is seen more commonly in patient's with psoriasis

REFERENCES

1. Henseler T, Christophers E. Disease concomitance in psoriasis. J Am Acad Dermatol. 1995;32:982-6.
2. Bjorksten B, Gustavson KH, Eriksson B. Recurrent multifocal osteomyelitis and pustulosis palmoplantaris. J Paediatr. 1978;93:227-31.
3. Prodanovich S, Kirsner RS, Kravetz JD, Ma F, Martinez L, Federman DG. Association of psoriasis with coronary artery, cerebrovascular, and peripheral vascular diseases and mortality. Archives of Dermatology. 2009;145(6):700-3.
4. Najarian DJ, Gottlieb AB. Connections between psoriasis and Crohn's disease. J Am Acad Dermatol. 2003;48:805-21.
5. Margolis D, Bilker W, Hennessy S, et al. The risk of malignancy associated with psoriasis. Arch Dermatol. 2001;137:778-83.
6. Johnston A, Arnadottir S. Obesity in psoriasis: Leptin and resistin as mediators of cutaneous inflammation. Br J Dermatol. 2008;159:342-50.
7. Garrets M. Psoriasiform dermatosis associated with bizarre metabolic abnormalities. Proc R Soc Med. 1961;54:220-3.

Chapter 12

Metabolic Syndrome and Psoriasis

Metabolic syndrome (Met S) is a clustering of risk factors comprising of abdominal obesity, dyslipidemia, elevated blood pressure and abnormal glucose tolerance. The prevalence of Met S has been increasing in the last few years throughout the world. Psoriasis has consistently been associated with metabolic syndrome as well as its various components. However, the association is no longer limited to psoriasis alone. Various dermatological conditions, such as lichen planus, androgenetic alopecia, systemic lupus erythematosus, skin tags, acanthosis nigricans and even cutaneous malignancies have also been found to be associated with this syndrome. Though chronic inflammation is thought to be the bridging link, the role of oxidative stress and endocrine abnormalities has recently been proposed in bringing them together.[1]

The mortality risk of coronary artery disease is around three times more in patients of metabolic syndrome. Different groups such as National Cholesterol Education Program's Adult Treatment Panel III, World Health Organization and the European Group on Insulin Resistance, agree on the essential components of metabolic syndrome with minor differences in details and criteria. Out of all these, the most commonly worldwide used criterion is the one proposed by National Cholesterol Education Program's ATP III. It requires the presence of at least three of the following: Abdominal obesity: Waist circumference: ≥102 cm in men or ≥88 cm in women, elevated triglycerides: ≥150 mg/dL, reduced high-density lipoprotein (HDL) cholesterol: <40 mg/dL for men, <50 mg/dL for women, elevated blood pressure: ≥130 mmHg systolic or ≥85 mmHg diastolic and elevated fasting blood glucose: ≥110 mg/dL. It has been found that the cardiovascular risk conferred by metabolic syndrome is higher than the individual components and hence it is important to study the association of diseases with metabolic syndrome as a whole.[2] Over the past few decades, there has been an alarming increase in the prevalence of metabolic syndrome in industrialized as well as in developing nations in the world. Approximately, one-third of the adult population in developed countries can be categorized as having metabolic syndrome by different definitions. In India, the incidence of metabolic syndrome was found to be 18.3% in a large-scale trial in Chennai in 2006. Recent evidence suggests that various dermatological diseases are associated with metabolic sydrome and/or its components. The diseases include psoriasis, androgenetic alopecia (AGA), acanthosis nigricans (AN), skin tags, lichen planus (LP), acne inversa (AI), systemic lupus erythematosus (SLE) and even skin cancer. As the exact mechanism by which these disorders are related to metabolic syndrome is yet to be explained, molecular studies are needed to further our understanding on this association.[3]

Among all cutaneous disorders, psoriasis has been found to be having the strongest association with Met S as well as its individual components. In view of increasing literature about it being a systemic disease, it is now classified as an immune-mediated inflammatory disease (IMID) of the skin. It is possible that the first event that occurs is the onset of psoriasis, followed by lifestyle changes and depression associated with smoking or overeating. These habits can lead to the metabolic syndrome. The National Psoriasis Foundation has found a moderate to large negative impact of the disease on the quality of life of patients, with an alteration of everyday activities. Impaired health-related quality of life may lead to unhealthy lifestyle behaviors, such as smoking, alcohol consumption, decreased physical activity and obesity, which are independent risk factors for cardiovascular diseases. In contrast, it is possible that obesity favors psoriasis in predisposed individuals because of the proinflammatory state and release of inflammatory mediators, such as adipocytokines.

Chronic inflammation is thought to be the bridging link between psoriasis and metabolic syndrome. Inflammatory markers, such as Th1 cytokines (intercellular adhesion molecule-1, TNF-α) play a role in the pathogenesis of psoriasis, Met S, obesity, atherosclerosis and myocardial infarction. Cytokines of the Th1 pathway (interferon-γ, IL-2, IL-12, and TNF-α) predominate in psoriatic and atherosclerotic plaques. Adhesion molecules including intercellular adhesion molecule-1 (ICAM-1) and vascular cell adhesion molecule (VCAM-1) are upregulated in psoriasis promoting adhesion of inflammatory cells to vascular endothelium, which in turn promote the formation of atherosclerotic plaques and obesity-related insulin resistance by oxidation of low-density lipoproteins in vessel wall. Proinflammatory glycoproteins like osteopontin, peptide hormones like leptin and adiponectin and other markers like homocysteine and CRP have also been implicated in bringing the two conditions together. Dysregulation of T-cell interactions and overexpression of proinflammatory cytokines lead to the hyperproliferaton of keratinocytes and activation of neutrophils in the epidermis. This results in chronic T-cell activation, resulting in a persistent cycle of inflammation and formation of psoriatic plaques. Vascular endothelial growth factor-induced angiogenesis, found both in psoriasis and atherosclerosis, has also been proposed as a common link between the two conditions. Several drugs used to treat psoriasis and/or psoriatic arthritis also have effects on the endothelium and may result in vascular complications.

After the initial work done by McDonald and Calabresi in1978, several hundred studies have been conducted worldwide to examine the association between psoriasis and cardiovascular diseases. Individual components of metabolic syndrome, such as obesity, hypertension, dyslipidemia and insulin resistance have been proved beyond doubt to be the comorbidities of psoriasis. Psoriatics have 2–3 fold higher risk of developing metabolic syndrome as compared to age-matched controls. The incidence of metabolic syndrome is significantly higher in psoriatics after the age of 40. One Indian study, however, found the highest prevalence of metabolic syndrome in the age group 18–30. This association has been found regardless of the gender of the patient, except in a single study showing definite female preponderance. Much work has been done to correlate the severity of psoriasis and risk of developing metabolic syndrome and its complications. Psoriatic patients with a higher psoriasis area severity index score are more likely to develop metabolic syndrome although the claim has been refuted by others. It has also been observed that psoriasis patients with metabolic syndrome had a longer disease duration compared with psoriatics without metabolic syndrome.[4,5]

The worldwide prevalence of psoriasis among children is approximately 1%. Even in children, it has been found to be associated with obesity, hyperlipidemia, diabetes and a statistically significant increased rate of the metabolic syndrome when compared with age-

and gender-matched controls. Moreover, there is evidence that treatment of psoriasis has a beneficial effect on the treatment outcome of concomitant vascular diseases. Methotrexate reduces the risk of major cardiovascular events in patients with psoriasis, psoriatic arthritis and rheumatoid arthritis compared to untreated controls. Therapy with TNF-α antagonists has been found to reduce levels of CRP, particularly in obese patients and to improve insulin sensitivity in patients with coexisting diabetes.[6]

In spite of so many reported studies signifying the association between psoriasis and metabolic syndrome, many study groups worldwide have failed to find any causal association between the two conditions.

Psoriasis is a chronic inflammatory skin disorder in which proinflammatory cytokines including IL-6 and TNF-α increase both locally and systematically. It is thought that chronic inflammation results in metabolic diseases and proinflammatory cytokines give rise to the development of atherogenesis, peripheral insulin resistance, hypertension and type 2 diabetes. Hypertension, diabetes mellitus and metabolic syndrome are significantly more common in psoriatic patients than controls. Therefore, all dermatologists should be aware of metabolic syndrome as individual components of metabolic syndrome might be associated with psoriasis during the course of this disease. Recent studies showed that psoriasis is associated with metabolic disorders, such as hypertension, type II diabetes mellitus (DM), dyslipidemia, abdominal obesity, insulin resistance and cardiac disorders and the risk of metabolic syndrome is increased in patients with psoriasis. Sommer et al. in their study reported that there is a significant association between psoriasis and type II DM, hypertension, hyperlipidemia and coronary artery disease and MS is increased by twofolds in a study they conducted in 581 patients.[7] Other studies showed an increased frequency of ischemic heart disease, DM, hypertension and dyslipidemia in patients with psoriasis when compared to controls. Gisondi et al. found increased prevalence of hypertrygliceridemia and MS in psoriasis patients compared to controls, but they did not find any difference between psoriasis patients and controls with respect to low levels of HDL, DM and hypertension.[8] Farshchian et al. failed to demonstrate any difference between psoriasis patients and controls with regard to fasting blood glucose, triglyceride, cholesterol, HDL, LDL and VLDL levels. Cohen et al. also demonstrated that the association between psoriasis and MS was pronounced after the age of 50. However, Nisa and Qazi observed the higher prevalence of MS in psoriasis patients in the age group 18–30.[9]

It is thus obvious that psoriasis predisposes to the development of DM, hypertension and metabolic syndrome and psoriasis increases the prevalence of metabolic syndrome by 3-fold. Therefore, it is recommended to evaluate psoriasis patients for the presence of metabolic diseases which may interfere with the patient's health for the rest of their living.

Points to Remember

- Metabolic syndrome is a more common association with psoriasis than earlier thought
- Weight reduction, low-calorie intake, intake of PUFAs and increased antioxidant intake has been found to decrease the severity of psoriasis

REFERENCES

1. Azfar R, S Gelfand JM. Psoriasis and metabolic disease: epidemiology and pathophysiology. Curr Opin Rheumatol. 2008;20(4):416-22.
2. Kimball AB, Gladman D, Gelfand JM, Gordon K, Horn EJ, Korman NJ, et al. National Psoriasis Foundation. National Psoriasis Foundation clinical consensus on psoriasis comorbidities and recommendations for screening. J Am Acad Dermatol. 2008;58(6):1031-42.
3. Neimann AL, Shin DB, Wang X, Margolis DJ, Troxel AB, Gelfand JM. Prevalence of cardiovascular risk factors in patients with psoriasis. J Am Acad Dermatol. 2006;55(5):829-35.
4. Gelfand JM, Neimann AL, Shin DB, Wang X, Margolis DJ, Troxel AB. "Risk of Myocardial Infarction in Patients with Psoriasis. "JAMA. 2006;292(14):1735-41.
5. Mallbris L, Akre O, Granath F. Increased risk for cardiovascular mortality in psoriasis inpatients but not in outpatients. Eur J Epidemiol. 2004;19:225-30.
6. Henseler T, Christophers E. Disease concomitance in psoriasis. J Am Acad Dermatol. 1995;32:982-6.
7. Sommer DM, Jenisch S, Suchan M, Christophers E, Weichenthal M. Increased prevalence of the metabolic syndrome in patients with moderate to severe psoriasis. Arch Dermatol Res. 2006;298(7):321-81.
8. Gisondi P, Tessai G, Conti A. Prevalance of metabolic syndrome in patients with psoriasis: A hospital based case-control study. Br J Dermatol. 2007;157:68-73.
9. Nisa N, Qazi MA. Prevalence of metabolic syndrome in patients with psoriasis. Indian J Dermatol Venereol Leprol. 2010;76(6):662-5.

Chapter

13 Psoriatic Arthritis

Psoriatic arthritis (arthritis psoriatica, arthropathic psoriasis or psoriatic arthropathy) is a type of seronegative inflammatory arthritis that develops in up to 30% of people with psoriasis. Psoriatic arthritis is said to be a seronegative spondyloarthropathy, associated with psoriasis of the skin and/or nails, with usually a negative serological test for rheumatoid factor and the absence of rheumatoid nodules.[1]

Estimation of the population prevalence of psoriatic arthritis is difficult and highly variable, depending on the study. The prevalence of arthritis among psoriatics has been estimated at 2.6–7%. However, a Scandinavian study revealed arthritis in 30% and in the USA, 23% of psoriatics. It may predate, occur concurrently or follow psoriasis. The nail disease is more frequent in cases with arthritis. In general there is no relationship between the extent and severity of psoriasis and psoriatic arthritis, which is more common in patients with generalized pustular psoriasis and erythrodermic psoriasis.[2] The age of onset for psoriatic arthritis has been found to be later than that for psoriasis vulgaris.

Psoriatic arthritis is a T-cell mediated disorder as intra-articular clonal expansion of CD8-expressing T cells have been observed, but the putative antigens remain elusive. A specific association with HLA-B27, Cw6, B13, B17 and DR13 has been reported as has familial clustering. Increased immunoreactivity to streptococcal antigens has been reported in sera of these patients. An increased prevalence of psoriatic arthritis has been reported in HIV and hepatitis C infection and antibodies to enterobacterial antigens are also recorded.[3]

How does psoriatic arthritis present clinically?

The common symptoms of psoriatic arthritis include the following:

- Pain, swelling, or stiffness in one or more joints.
- Tender joints which are red or warm to the touch.
- Sausage-like swelling in the fingers or toes, known as dactylitis.
- Pain in and around the feet and ankles, especially tendinitis in the Achilles tendon or Plantar fasciitis in the sole of the foot.
- Pain in the area of the sacrum (the lower back).

Factors that contribute to a diagnosis of psoriatic arthritis include:

- Psoriasis in the patient, or a family history of psoriasis or psoriatic arthritis.
- A negative test result for rheumatoid factor.
- Arthritis involving the distal interphalangeal joint of hand, which is not seen in rheumatoid arthritis.
- Ridging or pitting of fingernails or toenails, which is associated with psoriasis and psoriatic arthritis.
- X-ray evidence of joint changes.

Other symptoms that are more typical of psoriatic arthritis than other forms of arthritis include dactylitis (sausage-like swelling of the fingers or toes), inflammation of the Achilles tendon (at the back of the heel) or the Plantar fascia (bottom of the feet).[4]

CLASSIFICATION[5]

There are five main types of psoriatic arthritis (Moll and Wright's classification) (Figs 13.1 to 13.6):

- *Asymmetric:* This type affects around 70% of patients and is generally mild. This type does not occur in the same joints on both sides of the body and usually involves fewer than 3 joints. It is the most common form and often overlooked.
- *Symmetric:* This type accounts for around 25% of cases and affects joints on both sides of the body simultaneously. This type is most similar to rheumatoid arthritis and is disabling in around 50% of all cases.
- *Arthritis mutilans:* Affects less than 5% of patients and is a severe, deforming and destructive arthritis. This condition can progress over months or years causing severe joint damage. Arthritis mutilans has also been called chronic absorptive arthritis and may be seen in rheumatoid arthritis as well.
- *Spondylitis:* This type is characterised by stiffness of the spine or neck, but can also affect the hands and feet, in a similar fashion to symmetric arthritis.
- *Predominant distal interphalangeal arthritis:* This type of psoriatic arthritis is found in about 5% of patients and is characterized by inflammation and stiffness in the joints nearest to the ends of the fingers and toes. Nail changes are often marked.

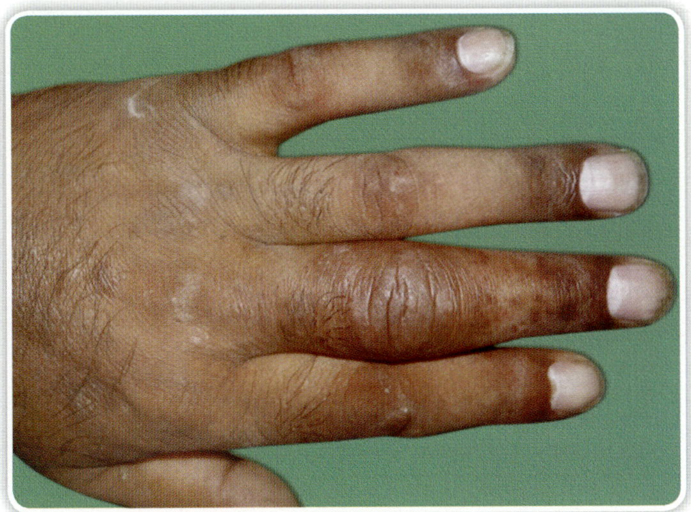

FIG. 13.1: Dactylitis (painful swollen middle finger) in a patient of psoriatic arthritis

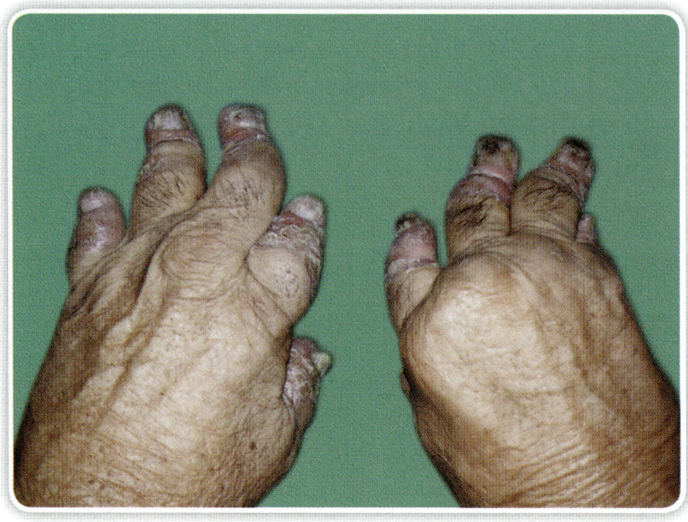

FIG. 13.2: Arthritis mutilans in an elderly patient with a long duration of psoriasis

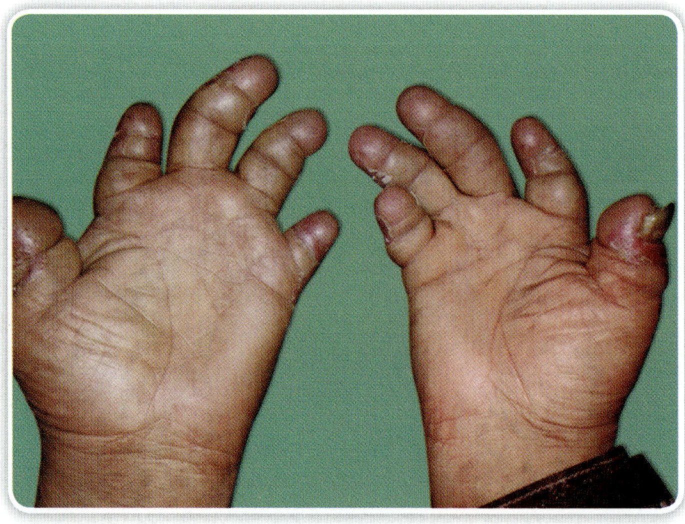

FIG. 13.3: Volar aspect of the same patient with arthritis mutilans. Note the characteristic resorption of digits and associated psoriatic changes involving nails and phalanges

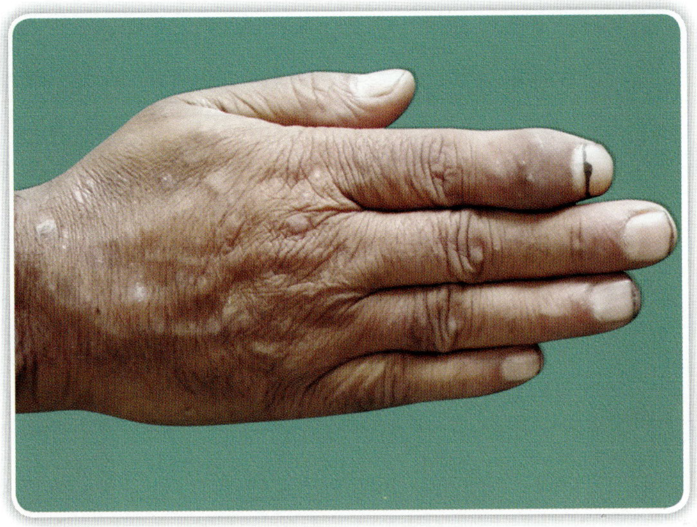

FIG. 13.4: Distal interphalangeal joint (right index finger) involvement in psoriatic arthritis

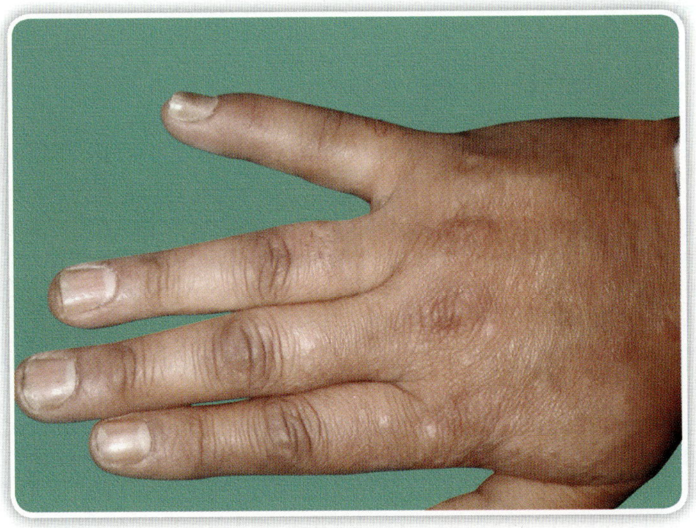

FIG. 13.5: Dactylitis involving the right little finger

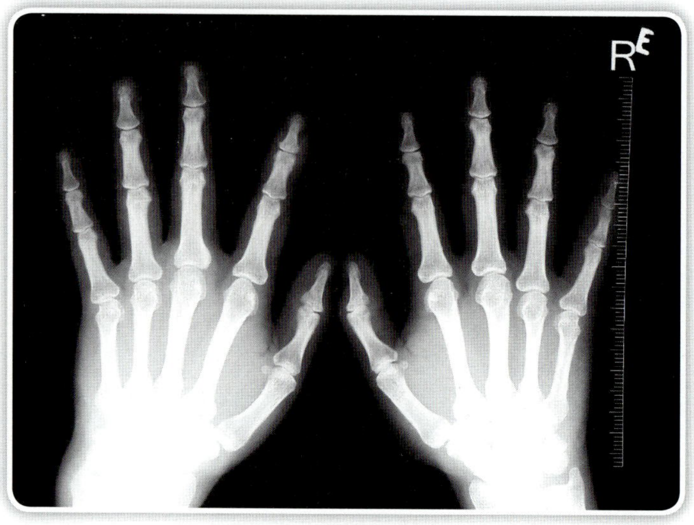

FIG. 13.6: X-ray of hands showing joint-space narrowing and terminal phalangeal resorption

Classification of Psoriatic Arthritis

The classification criteria for psoriatic arthritis **(CASPAR)** consist of established inflammatory articular disease with at least 3 points from the following features:[6]

- Current psoriasis (assigned a score of 2)
- A history of psoriasis (in the absence of current psoriasis; assigned a score of 1)
- A family history of psoriasis (in the absence of current psoriasis and history of psoriasis; assigned a score of 1)
- Dactylitis (assigned a score of 1)
- Juxta-articular new-bone formation (assigned a score of 1)
- Rheumatoid factor negativity (assigned a score of 1)
- Nail dystrophy (assigned a score of 1)

LABORATORY FINDINGS[7]

No specific diagnostic tests are available for psoriatic arthritis. The most characteristic laboratory abnormalities in patients with this condition are as follows:

- Elevation of the erythrocyte sedimentation rate (ESR) and C-reactive protein levels.
- Negative rheumatoid factor in 91–95% of patients.
- In 10–20% of patients with generalized skin disease, the serum uric acid concentration may be increased.
- Low levels of circulating immune complexes have been detected in 56% of patients
- Serum immunoglobulin A levels are increased in two thirds of patients.
- Synovial fluid is inflammatory, with cell counts ranging from 5000 to 15,000/μL and with more than 50% of cells being polymorphonuclear leukocytes; complement levels are either within reference ranges or increased and glucose levels are within reference ranges.

RADIOGRAPHIC STUDIES[8]

Radiologic features have helped to distinguish psoriatic arthritis from other causes of polyarthritis. The changes may be indistinguishable from those of rheumatoid arthritis. In general, the common subtypes of psoriatic arthritis, such as asymmetrical oligoarthritis and symmetrical polyarthritis, tend to result in only mild erosive disease. Early bony erosions occur at the cartilaginous edge and cartilage is initially preserved, with maintenance of a normal joint space.

The following radiographic abnormalities are suggestive of psoriatic arthritis:

- Pencil-in-cup deformity
- Joint-space narrowing in the interphalangeal joints, possibly with ankylosis
- Increased joint space in the interphalangeal joints as a result of destruction
- Fluffy periostitis
- Bilateral, asymmetrical, fusiform soft-tissue swelling
- Unilateral or symmetrical sacroiliitis
- Large, nonmarginal, unilateral, asymmetrical syndesmophytes (intervertebral bony bridges) in the cervical, thoracic, and lumbar spine, often sparing some of the segments.

MAGNETIC RESONANCE IMAGING STUDIES[9]

- MRI is particularly sensitive for detecting sacroiliitic synovitis, enthesitis, and erosions. It can also be used with gadolinium to increase sensitivity
- MRI may show inflammation in the small joints of the hands, involving the collateral ligaments and soft tissues around the joint capsule, a finding not seen in persons with rheumatoid arthritis.[7]

TREATMENTS[10-12]

Treatment follows the general lines of management of inflammatory polyarthritis and is best supervised by a rheumatologist. The underlying process in psoriatic arthritis is inflammation; therefore treatments are directed at reducing and controlling inflammation. Milder cases of psoriatic arthitis may be treated with NSAIDS alone; however, there is a trend towards earlier use of disease-modifying antirheumatic drugs or biological response modifiers to prevent irreversible joint destruction.

Nonsteroidal Anti-inflammatory Drugs

Nonsteroidal anti-inflammatory drugs (NSAIDs), such as ibuprofen and naproxen followed by more potent NSAIDs like diclofenac, indomethacin and etodolac are the agents which are first used for psoriatic arthritis. NSAIDs however, irritate the stomach and intestine and their long-term use can lead to gastrointestinal bleeding. Other potential adverse effects include damage to the kidneys and cardiovascular system.

Disease-modifying Anti-rheumatic Drugs

This class of drugs helps to limit the amount of joint damage that occurs in psoriatic arthritis, besides reducing pain and inflammation. Most, disease-modifying antirheumatic drugs (DMARDs) act slowly and may take weeks or even months to take full effect. Drugs, such as methotrexate or leflunomide are commonly prescribed; other DMARDS used to treat psoriatic arthritis include cyclosporin, azathioprine and sulfasalazine. Methotrexate is the most widely used and most effective agent for psoriatic arthritis, as it is effective for the skin lesions as well. A dose of 7.5–15 mg/week has been found to be superior to placebo in various studies. Ciclosporin is probably less effective than methotrexate for the treatment of psoriatic arthritis. Sulfasalazine has been found to have a small beneficial effect on peripheral synovitis and pain and despite earlier encouraging results, it has not been found to be an effective agent. These immunosuppressant drugs can also reduce psoriasis skin symptoms but can lead to hepatic and renal complications and lead to an increased risk of serious infections. The clinical subgroups of axial involvement associated with HLA-B27 has a relatively poor response to treatment.

Gold salts (oral auranofin) and intramuscular sodium thiomalate are used to treat psoriatic arthritis. Sodium thiomalate appears to be the better of the two, but less effective than methotrexate. The disadvantage of the use of gold salts is the occasional exacerbation of skin lesions of psoriasis.

Leflunomide (a pyrimidine synthesis inhibitor), effective for rheumatoid arthritis has been found to be effective for psoriatic arthritis in both short term (3 months) and long term (2 years) in a longitudinal study of eight patients. It is used in a dose of 10–20 mg/day after a loading dose of 100 mg.

Biological Response Modifiers for Psoriatic Arthritis

Recently, a new class of therapeutics called biological response modifiers or biologics has been developed using recombinant DNA technology. Biologic medications are derived from living cells cultured in a laboratory. Different from the traditional DMARDS that affect the entire immune system, biologics target specific parts of the immune system. They are given by injection or intravenous (IV) infusion.

Biologics prescribed for psoriatic arthritis are TNF-α inhibitors, including infliximab, etanercept, golimumab and adalimumab.

Biologics may increase the risk of minor and serious infections. More rarely, they may be associated with nervous system disorders, blood disorders or certain types of cancer.

OTHER TREATMENTS

Intra-articular joint injections with corticosteroids in cases where one joint is severely affected. In psoriatic arthritis, patients, with severe joint damage orthopedic surgery may be considered to correct joint destruction, usually with use of a joint replacement. Surgery is effective for pain alleviation, correcting joint disfigurement and reinforcing joint usefulness and strength.

Surgical Treatment Modalities for Psoriatic Arthritis

- Arthroscopic synovectomy has been found to be effective in treating severe, chronic, monoarticular synovitis
- Joint replacement and reconstructive therapy are occasionally necessary
- Patients with severe pain or with significant contractures may be referred for possible surgical intervention; however, high rates of recurrence of joint contractures have been noted after surgical release, especially in the hand
- Hip and knee joint replacements have been successful
- Arthrodesis and arthroplasty have also been used on joints, such as the proximal interphalangeal joint of the thumb
- For arthritis mutilans, surgical intervention is usually directed towards salvage of the hand. A combination of arthrodesis, arthroplasty and bone grafts to lengthen the digits may be used.

The rehabilitation treatment program for patients with psoriatic arthritis should be individualized and should be started early in the disease process, to decrease the morbidity associated with psoriatic arthritis.

Points to Remember

- ❖ Psoriatic arthritis is seen in 10–30% of patients with psoriasis. There is confusion whether it is an association or comorbidity or a separate disease
- ❖ Involvement of distal interphalangeal joint, enthesitis, plantar fasciitis and Achilles-tendinitis is characteristic of psoriatic arthritis
- ❖ Assymetrical oligoarthritis is the most common type of psoriatic arthritis

REFERENCES

1. Amherd-Hoekstra A, Näher H, Lorenz HM, Enk AH. "Psoriatic arthritis: A review." Journal of the German Society of Dermatology. 2010:8(5):332-9.
2. Zachariae H, Zachariae R, Blomqvist K, et al. Quality of life and prevalence of arthritis reported by 5795 members of the Nordic Psoriasis Associations. Data from the Nordic Quality of Life study. Acta Derma Venereol. 2002;82:108-13.
3. Lapadula G, Iannone F, Covelli M, et al. Anti-Enterobacteria antibodies in psoriatic arthritis. Clin Exp Rheumatol. 1992;10:461-6.
4. Baker H, Golden DN, Thompson M. Psoriasis and arthritis. Ann Intern Med. 1963;58:909-25.
5. Moll JMH, Wright V. Posriatic arthritis. Semin Arthritis Rheum. 1973;3:55-78.
6. Taylor W, Gladman D, Helliwell P, Marchesoni A, Mease P, Mielants H. Classification criteria for psoriatic arthritis: Development of new criteria from a large international study. Arthritis Rheum. 2006;54(8):2665-73.
7. Sherman M. Psoriatic arthritis: Observations on the clinical, roentgenographic and pathologic changes. J Bone Joint Surg Sm. 1952;34:831-52.
8. Avila R, Pugh DG, Slocumb CH, et al. Psoriatic arthritis: A roentgenologic study. Radiology. 1960;75:691-702.
9. Marzo-Ortega H, Tanner SF, Rhodes LA. Magnetic resonance imaging in the assessment of metacarpophalangeal joint disease in early psoriatic and rheumatoid arthritis. Scan J Rheumatol. 2009;38:79-83.

10. Fitzgerald O, Winchester R. Psoriatic arthritis: From pathogenesis to therapy. Arthritis Res Ther. 2009;11(1):214.
11. Griffiths CEM. Therapy for psoriatic arthritis: Sometimes a conflict for psoriasis. Br J Rheumatol. 1997;36: 409-10.
12. McInnes IB, Kavanaugh A, Gottlieb AB, Puig L, Rahman P, Ritchlin C, et al. Efficacy and safety of ustekinumab in patients with active psoriatic arthritis: 1 year results of the phase 3, multicentre, double-blind, placebo-controlled PSUMMIT 1 trial. Lancet. 2013;382(9894):780-9.

Chapter

14 Associations of Psoriasis

Rather than being limited to the skin, psoriasis is now believed to be a systemic immune-mediated inflammatory disease with several disease associations. There are several associations of psoriasis including arthritis, immunobullous disorders, vitiligo, metabolic syndrome and synovitis, acne, pustulosis, hyperostosis and osteitis (SAPHO) syndrome. Arthritis is the most common association first recognized by Jean Louis Alibert in 1818. In 1973, Moll and Wright clearly defined psoriatic arthritis (PsA) as a distinct entity under seronegative spondyloarthropathies and gave simple criteria for its diagnosis which include an inflammatory arthritis (peripheral arthritis and/or sacroiliitis or spondylitis), presence of psoriasis, absence (usually) of serological tests for rheumatoid factor. They also described its five main clinical patterns viz: distal interphalangeal (DIP) arthritis, arthritis mutilans (destructive), symmetric polyarthritis, asymmetric oligoarthritis and spondyloarthropathy. Other manifestations of PsA include enthesitis, tendonitis, fasciitis and dactylitis.[1,2]

The incidence of PsA is estimated to range from 7% to 42% among all psoriasis patients. There are only few studies on PsA from India. The peak incidence of PsA has been reported in the fifth and sixth decades of life. In most of the studies from India, males outnumbered females unlike rheumatoid arthritis (RA) which is more common in females. But the literature from West suggests female preponderance. The most common pattern of PsA reported in Western literature is asymmetric oligoarticular arthritis. However, Ray et al. and Rajendran et al. found polyarticular pattern simulating rheumatoid arthritis (RA) as the most common pattern. Isolated DIP arthritis is uncommon and arthritis mutilans is rare. Psoriasis lesions precede the onset of arthritis in more than 70% cases. PsA usually appears within 10 years of the onset of psoriasis and the chances of development after 10 years are very low. Significant number of psoriasis patients (27.5%) have positive family history.

The most common clinical phenotype observed in PsA patients is the chronic plaque type which is otherwise also the most common clinical presentation. Nail changes are common in psoriasis patients having concurrent PsA occurring in around 70% patients. The most common findings observed are pitting, subungual hyperkeratosis, discoloration, ridging and thickening of the nail plate. HLA association has been studied in few studies. Ray et al. found positive association of HLA-A1 and -B17 with the peripheral psoriatic arthritis.[3]

Recently, the association of psoriasis with metabolic syndrome has gained considerable attention in literature. Large number of studies in western literature suggests association of psoriasis with metabolic syndrome comprising of obesity, heart disease, hyperglycemia, dyslipidemia and hypertension. It has been recognized to contribute to the mortality risk in this group of patients. There are very few Indian studies to elucidate the role of metabolic syndrome in Indian patients. There is evidence for association of several lifestyle factors including alcohol and smoking and other diseases with psoriasis. But it can be reliably confirmed by appropriate study designs (cohort studies) which will help to elucidate the true associations and disentangle the temporal sequence.[4]

Bullous pemphigoid and vitiligo are two autoimmune diseases reported to be associated with psoriasis. More than 50 cases have been reported in literature, with coexisting psoriasis and bullous pemphigoid. Vitiligo coexisting and co-localizing with psoriasis has been reported from India. Dhar et al. reported co-localization of vitiligo and psoriasis in a 9-year-old boy and concluded that, there could be structural similarities between anti stratum corneum antibodies and anti melanocyte antibodies and that a common neuropeptide might be responsible for co-habitation of vitiligo and psoriasis. Kaur et al. has reported vitiligo as the most common cutaneous disease (1.7%) found to be associated with psoriasis. In a retrospective study (1989–2003), Sandhu et al. noted presence of vitiligo in 38 out of 4700 total psoriasis patients seen over this period. There was no definite pattern of distribution; psoriasis and vitiligo were distributed separately in 18 (47.3%) patients, whereas overlapping pattern where psoriasis lesions partly or completely covered some of the vitiliginous patches and also occurred at nonvitiliginous sites were seen in 13 (34.2%) patients. They did not find increased incidence of concurrence of both diseases and the onset and course of the psoriasis and vitiligo were independent of each other. Psoriasis lesions occurred on vitiliginous areas and normal skin with equal frequency, with strict co-localization being an uncommon feature.[5,6]

Crohn's disease is seen seven times more often in psoriatic patients. This may be due to overlapping inflammatory pathways common in both conditions or be a side effect of some of the biological agents used in the management of psoriasis, such as infliximab and adalimumab.[7] Some authors postulate that psoriasis may be associated with an increased risk of cancer (nonmelanoma skin cancer); however, this could be a side effect of psoriasis treatments, including photochemotherapy.[8]

Psoriasis has been reported rarely to occur more frequently in certain metabolic disorders. These include gout, hypoparathyroidism, diabetes and metabolic syndrome. Hypocalcemia has been reported in association with severe and pustular forms of psoriasis, including certain syndromes and following thyroidectomy.[9]

Chronic, recurrent, multifocal osteomyelitis is an unusual, sterile, inflammatory entity of unknown cause characterized by pain and swelling in affected bones. Association with pustular and nonpustular forms of psoriasis has been reported. Closely related to this entity is the SAPHO syndrome (synovitis, acne, pustulosis, hyperostosis and osteitis) most frequently described in the radiological and rheumatological literature.[10]

Points to Remember

- There are several associations of psoriasis including arthritis, immunobullous disorders, vitiligo, metabolic syndrome and SAPHO syndrome. Arthritis is the most common association
- Metabolic syndrome has recently been found to be increasingly associated with psoriasis. Appropriate management of metabolic syndrome decreases the severity of psoriasis

REFERENCES

1. Krueger GKoo, Lebwohl J, Menter M, Stern A, Rolstad RST. The impact of psoriasis on quality of life: Results of a 1998 National Psoriasis Foundation patient-membership survey. Arch Dermatol. 2001;137(3):280-4.
2. Moll JMH, Wright V. Posriatic arthritis. Semin Arthritis Rheum. 1973;3:55-78.
3. Baker H, Golden DN, Thompson M. Psoriasis and arthritis. Ann Intern Med. 1963;58:909-25.
4. Shapiro J, Cohen AD, David M. The association between psoriasis, diabetes mellitus, and atherosclerosis in Israel: A case-control study. J Am Acad Dermatol. 2007;56(4):629- 34.
5. Wilczek A, Sticherling M. Concomitant psoriasis and bullous pemphigoid: Coincidence or pathogenic relationship? Int J Dermatol. 2006;45:1353-7.
6. Percivalle S, Piccino R, Caccialanza M. Concurrence of vitiligo and psoriasis: A simple coincidence? Clin Exp Dermatol. 2009;34:90-1.
7. Najarian DJ, Gottlieb AB. Connections between psoriasis and Crohn's disease. J Am Acad Dermatol. 2003;48:805-21.
8. Margolis D, Bilker W, Hennessy S, et al. The risk of malignancy associated with psoriasis. Arch Dermatol. 2001;137:778-83.
9. Henseler T, Christophers E. Disease concomitance in psoriasis. J Am Acad Dermatol. 1995;32(6):982-6.
10. Laxer RM, Shore AD, Manson D, et al. Chronic recurrent multifocal osteomyelitis and psoriasis: A report of a new association and review of related disorders. Semin Arthritis Rheum. 1988;17:260-70.

Chapter

15

Psychiatric Comorbidity in Psoriasis

Psoriasis produces significant adverse effects on the psychological and social aspects of life mainly because of its visibility. There are few studies from India addressing this aspect of the disease.

Rakhesh et al. studied 50 psoriasis patients aged more than 18 years assessing their clinical severity, physical and psychosocial disability and stress incurred by measuring psoriasis area severity index (PASI), psoriasis disability index (PDI) and psoriasis life stress inventory (PLSI), respectively. Among the physical and psychosocial factors investigated; daily activities, employment and treatment were most affected. They also concluded that psoriasis sufferers feel self-conscious, disturbed/inconvenienced by the shedding of the skin, live in a constant fear of relapse and avoid social interactions.

Gaikwad et al. in a study of 43 psoriasis patients found that their disease affected the social functioning, led to decreased work efficiency and subjective distress at work in more than half of the subjects. Around two-third patients consented that psoriasis has affected their interpersonal relationship resulting in stress in home environment. Sixty-seven percentage of the patients had psychiatric comorbidity. Mattoo et al. studied psychiatric morbidity in 103 psoriasis patients and 113 vitiligo patients at hospital settings in Chandigarh. The general health questionnaire (GHQ) assessed psychiatric morbidity rates at 33.63% and 24.7% for vitiligo and psoriasis, respectively. The ICD-10 psychiatric diagnoses in GHQ positive cases were adjustment disorder (56% vs 62%), depressive episode (22% vs 29%) and dysthymia (9% vs 4%) in vitiligo and psoriasis, respectively. The comprehensive psychopathological rating scale (CPRS) assessed that depression, anxiety and total psychopathology levels were similar in the two GHQ positive subgroups.[1-3]

So, these studies suggest that psoriasis leads to significant psychosocial disability in the patients and this facet of the disease should be addressed while managing any patient by means of psychological and behavior therapy.

REFERENCES

1. Rakesh SV, D'Souza M, Sahal A. Quality of life in psoriasis: A study from South India. Indian J Dermatol Venereol Leprol. 2008;74:600-6.
2. Mattoo SK, Handa S, Kaur I, Gupta N, Malhotra R. Psychiatric morbidity in psoriasis: Prevalence and correlates in India. German J Psychiatry. 2005;8:17-22.
3. Gupta MA, Gupta AK, Watteel GN. Perceived deprivation of social touch in psoriasis is associated with greater psychologic morbidity: an index of the stigma experience in dermatologic disorders. Cutis. 1999;61:339-42.

Chapter

16 Childhood Psoriasis

Psoriasis is a common genetically determined chronic inflammatory skin disease characterized by complex alteration in epidermal proliferation and differentiation. It exhibits a bimodal age distribution—childhood psoriasis that occurs before 18 years and adult psoriasis that occurs after 18 years. Psoriasis is not uncommon in childhood. The childhood psoriasis is a well-recognized entity; however, its true prevalence is not exactly known yet. Childhood psoriasis can be further classified as (i) congenital psoriasis, (ii) infantile psoriasis, (iii) psoriasis with early onset and (iv) pediatric psoriasis with psoriatic arthritis. Congenital psoriasis may be associated with a lower prevalence of a positive family history and a higher fraction of erythrodermic and pustular forms of the disease with a poorer prognosis. Infantile psoriasis usually has its onset within the 1st year of life and has got a better prognosis. The other subtypes have their onset during adolescence and teenage years.[1]

Psoriasis in children can be a life-changing disease with profound physical and psychosocial impact on the quality of life. Childhood psoriasis differs from that in adults in epidemiology, clinical features, treatment and long-term clinical and psychological outcome. Study of the disease in the pediatric age group is thus very important because of the psychological problems, dangers inherent to systemic therapies and alteration of the natural course of the disease by various factors.[2]

In a study conducted by Manoharan R and colleagues, in Tamil Nadu, a complete analysis of the out patient records of patients with psoriasis who had attended the dermatology out-patient department of their hospital for a period of 8 months between september 2011 and april 2012 was done. All the demographic details were collected and the age at presentation of the disease was also noted.

The incidence of childhood psoriasis that was observed in their study was 17.15%. The incidence of psoriasis in male and female children was thus observed to be 49.15% and 50.84% respectively in their study. The mean age of onset of childhood psoriasis in boys was observed to be 12.8 years and in girls, it was observed to be 13.8 years. The male female ratio was observed to be 1:1.03.[3]

Congenital psoriasis is very rare. Psoriasis is relatively uncommon in children. In approximately one-third of patients, psoriasis begins in the first two decades of life. Guttate psoriasis is the most common variant in children. Apart from the common forms, several other patterns of psoriasis occur in childhood. Interdigital tinea is uncommon in children and a toe cleft intertrigo may be psoriatic. Other flexural forms also occur. Facial psoriasis is seen more in children as compared to adults. A new variant known as psoriaform acral dermatitis is seen especially in children.[4]

Psoriasis is relatively uncommon but a burdensome disease in children. There are few epidemiological studies on childhood psoriasis. Infantile psoriasis is less defined as there is clinical overlap with other common dermatoses of this age group like atopic dermatitis and seborrhoeic dermatitis. Psoriasis in children has few peculiar features which have been consistently observed in studies on childhood psoriasis. Guttate psoriasis is more common, spontaneous remissions are relatively more common than in adults while relapses usually follow infections. Certain clinical variants like erythroderma, localized and generalized pustular psoriasis and arthropathy are uncommon.[5]

Western literature reports psoriasis prevalence to be around 0.71% in children. The only comprehensive prevalence analysis of juvenile psoriasis till date showed the prevalence in United Kingdom of about 0.6% in children aged 0–9 years and 1.4% in children aged 10–19 years. In a large series of 1262 psoriasis children from Australia, age of patients ranged from 1 month to 15 years, there was equal incidence in males and females, family history was present in a significant number of cases (71%), plaque type of psoriasis was the most common clinical phenotype (34%), facial involvement was common (38%) and infantile psoriasis presented as diaper rash commonly.[6]

In a study from South India done to evaluate the pattern of dermatoses in children, psoriasis accounted for 1.4% of the total skin patients presenting in an out patient department of a hospital over a period of one year. In India, the largest series on childhood psoriasis was reported by Kumar et al. They presented data of 419 children with psoriasis. Children accounted for 12.5% of total psoriasis patients over a period of 13 years. The age of onset ranged from 4 days to 14 years; male and female incidence was equal and plaque type psoriasis was the most common clinical presentation. Unlike the study by Morris et al. familial incidence was low (4.5%) and facial involvement was uncommon.[7]

Pediatric psoriasis consists of three age groups of psoriatic patients like infantile psoriasis, a self-limited disease of infancy; psoriasis with early onset and pediatric psoriasis with psoriatic arthritis. The varied clinical presentations in childhood include plaque-type, guttate, erythrodermic, napkin and nail-based disease. Like all forms of autoimmunity, susceptibility is likely genetic, but environmental triggers are required to initiate disease activity.[8]

The disease in children is more pruritic, common in girls and the lesions are relatively thinner, softer and less scaly. Plaque type is the most common form of disease, but certain clinical variants are rare in children like erythroderma, arthropathy and localized and generalized pustular psoriasis. Psoriasis in children is more frequently precipitated by infections and manifests as acute guttate psoriasis. However, Indian studies show that children manifest the established plaque type of disease more often, rather than the guttate variety. Facial involvement in children is a frequent observation in majority of the reports, which varies from 18 to 46%, whereas mucosal involvement has been rare in Indian children.[9]

A study from North India reported that extensors of the legs were the most common initial site affected (25% cases), followed by the scalp (20.7%). Classical plaque psoriasis was the most frequent clinical presentation (60.6%), followed by plantar psoriasis (12.8%). Nail involvement was observed in (31%) cases. Pitting was the most common nail change, followed by ridging and discoloration. Five children (1.1%) (three girls and two boys) had psoriatic arthropathy. Koebnerization was observed in 27.9% of patients.[10]

Another study showed that plaque psoriasis was the most common type (52.6%), followed by guttate psoriasis (25.5%), pustular psoriasis (10.9%) and psoriatic erythroderma (5.1%). Scalp was the most common initial site affected (50.3%), nail changes were found in 25.5%, but no mucosal involvement was observed (Figs 16.1 to 16.11).[11]

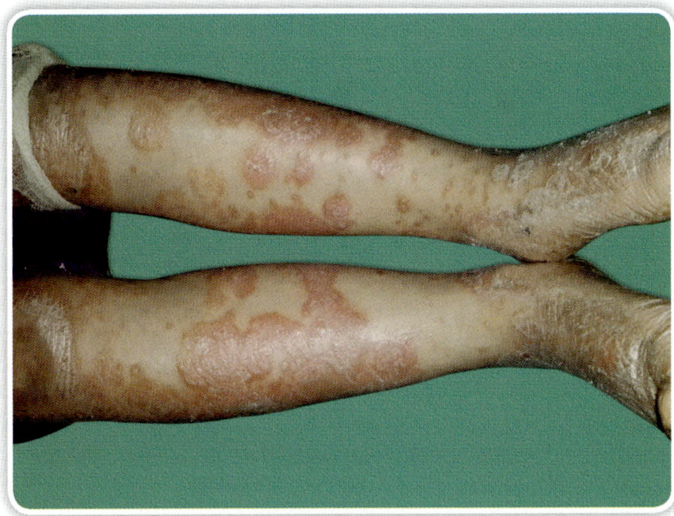

FIG. 16.1: Well-defined plaques of psoriasis vulgaris involving lower limbs in a young girl

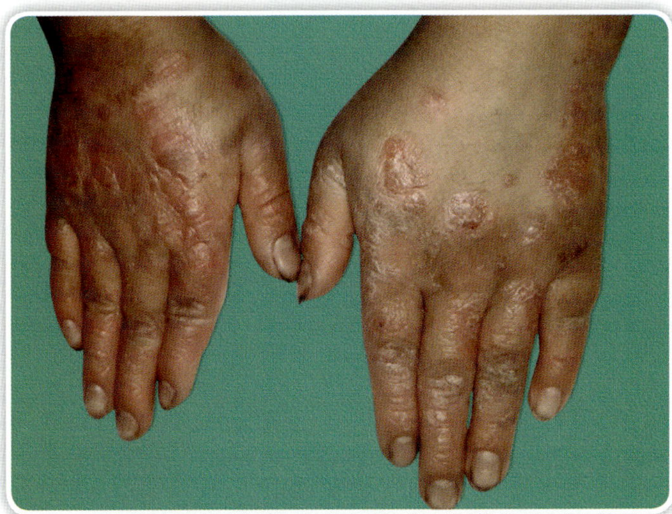

FIG. 16.2: Well-defined plaques of psoriasis vulgaris involving dorsa of both hands in the same patient

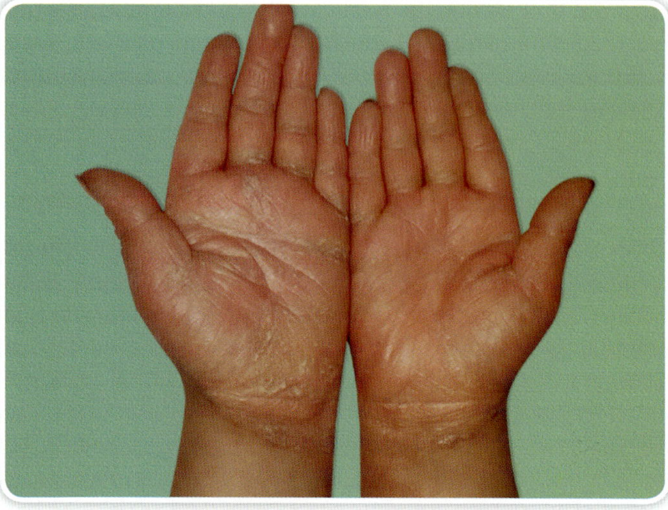

FIG. 16.3: Palmar leions in the same patient

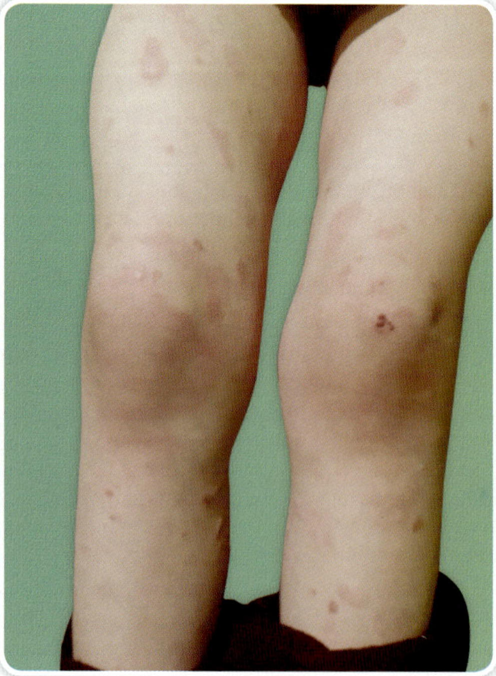

FIG. 16.4: Resolving psoriatic lesions in a young 7-year-old girl

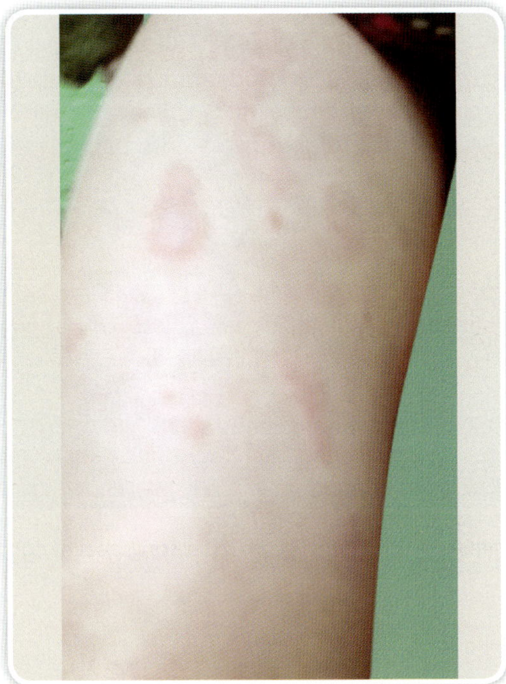

FIG. 16.5: Same patient showing resolving psoriatic lesions over trunk

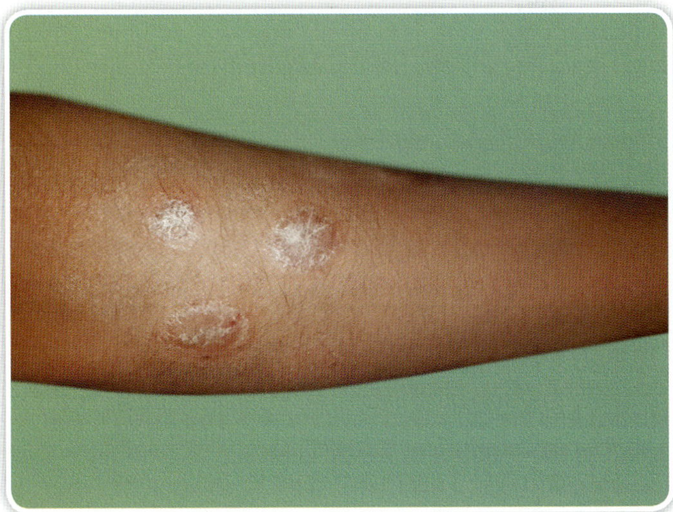

FIG. 16.6: Characteristic plaques of psoriasis over the extensor aspect of right arm in a young boy

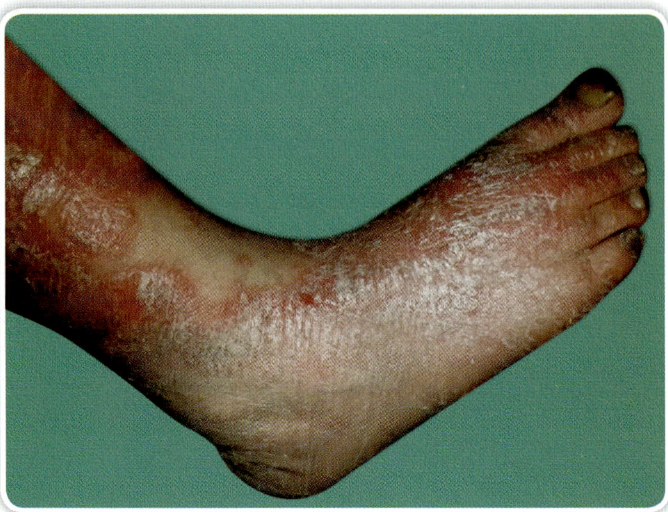

FIG. 16.7: Characteristic plaques of psoriasis over the extensor aspect of right lower limb in a young girl

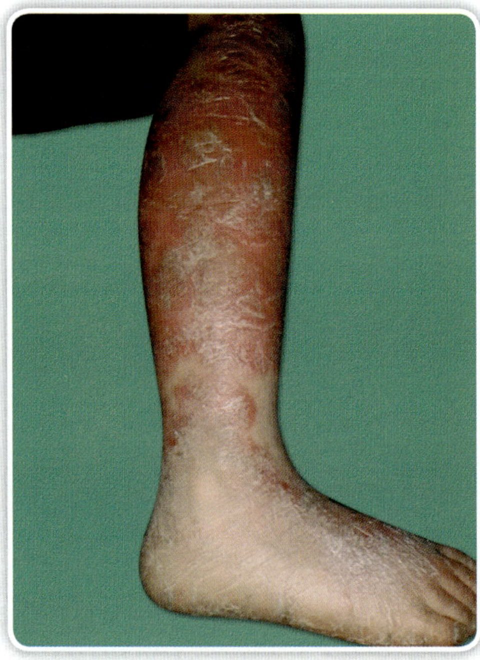

FIG. 16.8: Same patient showing closer view of characteristic plaques of psoriasis over the extensor aspect of right lower limb

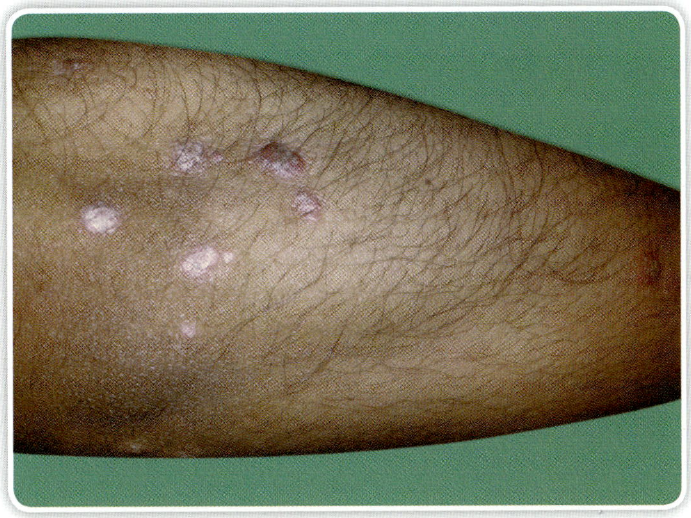

FIG. 16.9: Characteristic psoriatic plaques involving right forearm in a young boy

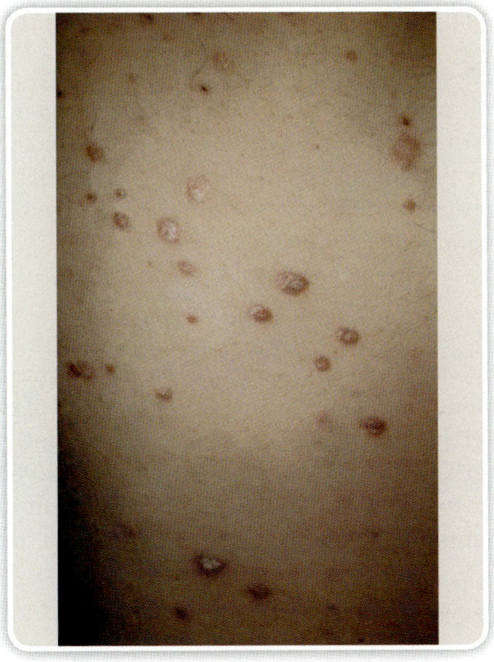

FIG. 16.10: Guttate psoriatic lesions over the back in a young girl

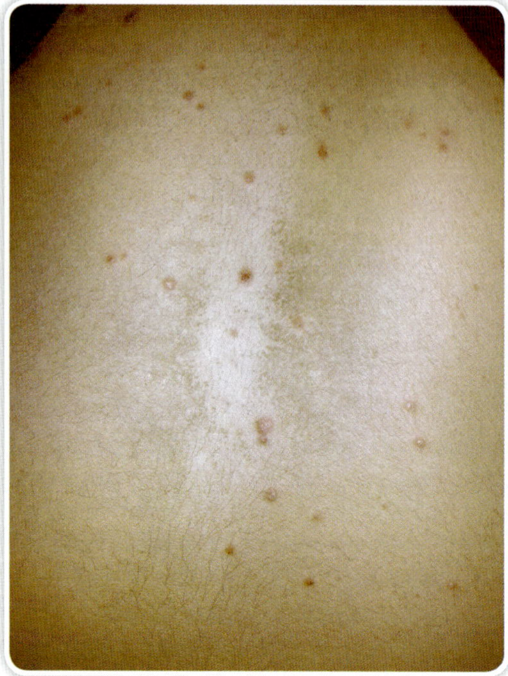

FIG. 16.11: Another patient showing guttate psoriatic lesions over the back.

MANAGEMENT STRATEGIES FOR CHILDHOOD PSORIASIS

Childhood psoriasis differs from that in adults in epidemiology, clinical features, treatment and long-term clinical and psychological outcome. The various treatment modalities which are used and have been investigated in childhood psoriasis include topical treatments, phototherapy and systemic therapies. The inflammatory nature of psoriasis has initiated study of the use of biological agents in children, which are characterized by targeted mode of action and hence a better safety profile.[12]

Topical Therapy

Psoriasis covering less than 5% of body surface area (BSA) can be managed in most patients with the use of topical agents alone. These agents are the cornerstone of treatment for most patients with psoriasis. Topical therapies however, do not always work for nail psoriasis even though they are easy to administer and readily available. Patients should be counselled to keep nails as short as possible, avoid manicures and prevent accumulation of any exogenous material under the nail. Any concomitant nail fungal infections should be treated appropriately.[13]

Role of Moisturizers

Moisturizers are complex mixtures of chemical agents specially designed to make the external layers of the skin softer and more pliable. They increase the skin's hydration by reducing evaporation. Moisturizers have a role in normalizing hyperproliferation and they exert anti-inflammatory effects by way of the physiologic lipids. An improved barrier function and hydration makes the epidermis less vulnerable to external trauma, thereby reducing the induction of Koebnerization. Pretreatment with emollients like mineral oil or vaseline augments the therapeutic efficacy of narrow-band ultraviolet-B therapy, possibly because it penetrates the intercellular space, producing an optical matching effect which enhances the UV transmission.[14]

Coal Tar

Coal tar is a complex and variable mixture of polycyclic aromatic hydrocarbons, phenols and heterocyclic compounds. It is among the by-products when coal is carbonized to coke or gasified to make coal gas. Coal tar is antiproliferative and can be used as ointment, cream or solution in concentrations ranging from 0.5 to 20%. Tar has been found to be safe and effective for childhood psoriasis, mainly for plaque type lesions. It can be used in combination with other medications like topical corticosteroids, salicylic acid and with UV irradiation. It is irritating on the face and flexures in children. Anthralin (dithranol) is a potent anti-inflammatory and antiproliferative agent used as "short-contact" or "minute" therapy, to reduce side effects like irritation and temporary perilesional staining of the skin. In an open study of 58 children aged 5–10 years treated with dithranol at concentrations up to 1%, remission was achieved in 47 (81%) patients.[15]

Emollients

An emollient is a humectant, lubricant and occluder. Occlusion provides a layer of oil on the skin surface, thus slowing down water loss. A humectant enhances the capacity of skin to hold water. A lubricant reduces friction when anything rubs against the skin. Emollients can have antipruritic, anti-inflammatory, rehydrant and skin barrier restorant properties as well. In simple terms, they reduce water loss, prevent the skin from drying out and create a barrier against the environment. Emollients are particularly useful in inflammatory and chronic plaque psoriasis as well as in acral psoriasis. In psoriasis, emollients offer relief from dryness, scaling and cracking of the skin and might also have an antiproliferative effect. Emollient monotherapy may be sufficient only in mild psoriasis. In most cases other adjuvants are required. Water-in-oil emollients have been shown to replace the requirement for daily use of corticosteroids. Some authors recommend a daily warm bath followed by liberal application of emollients together with one or two more moisturizing applications throughout the day. The use of emollients is associated with side effects such as irritant dermatitis, allergic contact dermatitis, stinging, cosmetic acne and dyspigmentation.[16]

Keratolytics

Topical keratolytics are agents that are applied on the skin to soften the keratin. They loosen and assist exfoliation of the skin cells. Keratolytics also help the skin to bind moisture and is useful in treating dry skin conditions. Perhaps the most widely used and oldest keratolytic agent known today, salicylic acid is available in concentrations ranging from 0.5% to 60% in a number of vehicles. It is particularly useful in thick plaque or scaly plaque psoriasis. In some patients salicylic acid may be useful as monotherapy. It can also be added to anthralin and zinc pastes to reduce the interaction between these two ingredients. Additionally, salicylic acid offers antioxidant properties to such preparations.

Application on large areas and in concentrations greater than 10% results in toxicity, especially in children. This manifests as oral mucosal burning, frontal headache, central nervous system symptoms, metabolic acidosis, tinnitus, nausea, vomiting and gastric symptoms. Salicylic acid may reduce the action of other therapies for psoriasis, including calcipotriene.[17]

Urea has both emollient and keratolytic properties. Furthermore, it can be combined with anthralin to improve its clinical efficacy. Urea combined with bifonazole is useful in the management of scalp psoriasis. It is used topically in concentrations of 5–25% in creams or lotions and up to 40% in nail preparations.[18]

Corticosteroids

Corticosteroids are perhaps the most widely used treatment for psoriasis worldwide. There are a number of corticosteroids available in the market that vary in their potency. The potency of earlier corticosteroids has been enhanced by chemical modification including halogenation, acetylation and methylation. The penetration of corticosteroids can be enhanced by using occlusive dressings or changing the base they are formulated in. Potent and very potent steroids are more useful than mild-to-moderate steroids in psoriasis.

Long-term effects of corticosteroid use include skin atrophy, telangiectasia, striae, purpura, iatrogenic Cushing's syndrome and hypothalamic-pituitary-adrenal (HPA) axis suppression. Since most studies are not conducted for long periods of time, the effects of tachyphylaxis are not well documented. Regimens to minimize the long-term effects are yet to be recognized.[19]

Vitamin D Analogues

These analogues (i.e. calcitriol, calcipotriene, tacalcitol) affect cellular differentiation and proliferation. Additionally, they regulate apoptosis and demonstrate an immunomodulatory effect. All vitamin D analogues allow a reduction in the duration and potency of other treatments. They are odorless and nonstaining and therefore cosmetically more acceptable than anthralin.

Calcitriol is an active metabolite of vitamin D, while as tacalcitol and calcipotriene are synthetic derivatives. All three cause hypercalcemia but are safe if used according to their respective dosage regimens. A model vitamin D analogue that has minor calcemic activity is yet to be developed. Other side effects include pruritus, burning, edema, peeling, dryness and erythema, which diminish with ongoing treatment.

Calcipotriene (also known as calcipotriol internationally) is slightly more effective than calcitriol and tacalcitol and is as effective as potent (but not ultrapotent) topical corticosteroids. A combination of calcipotriene with betamethasone reduces the long-term side effects of each ingredient by 1 year. Furthermore, since the combination has a low systemic absorption, the localized anti-inflammatory and immunoregulatory effect is higher than that of either of the individual drugs used separately. The combination is also available as a topical solution that is useful in the management of scalp psoriasis, delivering better efficacy and less irritation. In nail psoriasis, an application of calcipotriene may be used on its own or in combination with corticosteroids, particularly to manage subungual hyperkeratosis.

The concentration of calcipotriene used is 0.005% and it should not be applied more than twice daily. In children, the maximum dose is 50g for those aged 6–12 years and 75g for children above 12 years.

About 10% of patients using calcipotriene may notice a mild dermatitis on the face as a side effect. Calcipotriene also has a limited effect on calcium homeostasis as compared to calcitriol and tacalcitol. Calcitriol is better tolerated than calcipotriene in the treatment of easily irritated areas, such as the face, hairline and flexural areas.[20]

Tazarotene

This is a topical vitamin A derivative that is modified to tazarotenic acid through de-esterification in the skin. It appears to exert its beneficial effects by modulating cell proliferation and differentiation. Tazarotene can only be used once daily and therefore has limited use in monotherapy. It is less potent than vitamin D analogues and moderate or potent local corticosteroids. Tazarotene is used in patients in whom over 20% of the BSA is affected. The starting dose is a 0.05% cream or gel that can be increased to 0.1% as needed. It is normally used for 12 weeks at a time. The use of tazarotene for psoriasis may exacerbate acne. Since tazarotene is teratogenic, it should not be used by individuals who are pregnant or planning a pregnancy.[21]

Anthralin

This drug has been used in the treatment of psoriasis for over 80 years, but due to its staining properties, it is not a cosmetically acceptable agent. It demonstrates lower efficacy than topical corticosteroids and vitamin D derivatives as monotherapy. It is thought to exert its effects through its action on mitochondria. Currently, anthralin is used for the management of subacute and chronic plaque psoriasis in two ways—conventional and short-contact treatment. Conventional treatment is initiated with 0.1% anthralin ointment or paste that is applied sparingly to the lesions only for a few hours and then washed off. If irritation occurs, the strength and contact time must be reduced. The strength is gradually increased to 0.5% and even up to 1% and the contact period is extended overnight. Short-contact treatment involves applying anthralin to the lesion in strengths of 0.1–2% for up to 60 minutes daily and then washing it off.

Treatment should be continued until the psoriasis clears. Since anthralin causes skin irritation and staining of the skin, clothing and furniture, it is best used in day care centers or hospitals. In many cases it is combined with coal tar to reduce irritation. Furthermore, it can be combined with phototherapy for better results. Use of anthralin should be avoided on the face, skin flexures and genitals; hands should be washed thoroughly after use. Anthralin should not be used in acute or pustular psoriasis or applied onto inflamed skin. It is useful to inform patients that staining slowly disappears upon discontinuation of treatment.[22]

Corticosteroids still remain the mainstay topical treatment of psoriasis, as they have anti-inflammatory and antiproliferative properties and reduce erythema, scaling and pruritus. Topical corticosteroids are used in chronic plaque type psoriasis as monotherapy or in combination with topical treatments like calcipotriol and tazarotene. Lower-potency preparations are indicated for facial, genital and intertriginous skin areas, whereas thick hyperkeratotic areas, such as the palms and soles, require high-potency agents. Halobetasol cream 0.05% and clobetasol propionate emulsion 0.05% seem to be efficacious treatments in childhood plaque psoriasis. Reported side effects were relatively mild in the treatment period of 2 weeks. A case report described the use of hydrocortisone 1% ointment in a 2-year-old child with pustular psoriasis.[23]

Topical tacrolimus (0.03%, 0.1%) and pimecrolimus (1%) are nonsteroidal immunomodulating macrolactams which block the enzyme calcineurin, thereby inhibiting the production of IL-2 and subsequent T-cell activation and proliferation. In two nonrandomized clinical trials, treatment of facial and flexural psoriasis with tacrolimus 0.1% was evaluated in which all patients showed clearance after a treatment period varying from 2 to 30 days. Tacrolimus 0.1% was also used in one case report in which facial psoriasis cleared totally.[24]

Phototherapy is preferred in older children and adolescents with moderate to severe disease in which topical treatments have failed. Guttate and thin plaque type lesions respond best to phototherapy. NB-UVB shows good results in the treatment of plaque and guttate psoriasis in childhood and has comparatively milder side effects.[25]

SYSTEMIC AGENTS IN CHILDHOOD PSORIASIS

There is a paucity of studies on the use of systemic therapies in childhood psoriasis. Oral antibiotics have been tried due to the belief that streptococcal infection may exacerbate chronic plaque psoriasis, as well as induce guttate psoriasis, but the results of various studies have been equivocal. In an uncontrolled trial, 9 patients were treated with either 250 mg of penicillin or erythromycin 4 times per day for 10–14 days, with the addition of 300 mg of rifampicin, given per day for the last 5 days. 5 patients had clearance or near clearance of the skin lesions, 4 had moderate improvement and exacerbation of the disease was not noted in any patient. In another study, there was less than 50% clearance of lesions with the use of thiamphenicol (methyl-sulfonyl analogue of chloramphenicol, which is mainly used for the treatment of venereal infections). However, in a case series of 4 patients who were treated with erythromycin in a dose of 50 mg/kg/d for 2 weeks, the psoriatic lesions disappeared completely in all the patients. In an another case report, a patient with guttate psoriasis was treated with amoxicillin/clavulanic acid in a dose of 50 mg/kg/d, which cleared all lesions after 3 weeks. Other antibiotics which have been tried with variable results include phenoxymethylpenicillin, macrolide antibiotics (azithromycin, erythromycin) and intramuscular benzene penicillin. Several researchers recommend testing for perianal and pharyngeal streptococcal infection in any child presenting with acute guttate, pustular or plaque psoriasis and treating with oral antibiotics when cultures are positive.[26]

Various studies have advocated tonsillectomy to decrease the frequency of exacerbations and increase the remission rate in chronic plaque psoriasis, but it should not be routinely done. It has been suggested that chronic recalcitrant cases of childhood psoriasis with frequent acute exacerbations should be subjected to tonsillectomy. Improvement of psoriasis after tonsillectomy is associated with a decrease in the frequency of circulating T cells that recognize streptococcal determinants and homologous skin determinants.

Methotrexate (MTX), an antimetabolite agent is a folic acid analogue that reversibly inhibits dihydrofolate reductase, disrupting DNA synthesis, repair and replication of T and B lymphocytes. It posesses immunomodulatory and anti-inflammatory properties and has advantages of efficacy, affordability and convenient weekly oral dose. It is FDA approved for the use of adult severe psoriasis, but is used off label in pediatric psoriasis. In children, 0.2–0.4 mg/kg/week orally is recommended. Kumar et al.[27] in a case series of 7 children treated with methotrexate in a dose of 0.2–0.4 mg/kg/week for a mean of 38.8 months, reported disease control in approximately 2 months. Their ages and duration of disease varied from 3.5 to 16 years (mean 12.14 years). Psoriatic erythroderma was seen in three patients, generalized pustular psoriasis in two and recalcitrant psoriasis and psoriatic arthropathy in one each. MTX was given in a single weekly oral dose of 3.75–25 mg (mean 16.6 mg). The duration of treatment necessary to control the disease varied from 6 to 10 weeks (mean 7.9 weeks). Total duration of MTX therapy was from 31.2 to 46.4 weeks (mean 38.8 weeks). Posttherapy disease-free interval ranged between 14.4 and 16.8 weeks (mean 15.5 weeks). Follow-up after withdrawal of MTX was from 16 to 28 weeks (mean 22.3 weeks). Total cummulative MTX dose ranged from 390 to 960 mg (mean 683.6 mg). Methotrexate was tolerated by nearly all patients, with history of nausea and vomiting in three patients which was relieved by folic acid supplementation. In a review of 10 cases of childhood psoriasis treated with MTX, a complete clearance was noted in 20% cases, almost complete clearance in 60% cases and no response in 10% of cases. MTX was given at an initial dose of 0.03–0.24 mg/kg/wk and was increased according to the patient's response to 0.10–0.41 mg/kg/wk. The duration of treatment varied from 6 to 178 weeks. The side effects associated with the use of methotrexate are nausea, vomiting, diarrhoea, headache, hepatotoxicity, bone marrow suppression, interstitial pneumonitis, fetal death/malformation and photosenstivity.[28]

Acitretin is an aromatic retinoid that acts in psoriasis by its anti-inflammatory activity. Treatment should be initiated and maintained at dosages at or below 0.5–1 mg/kg/d to limit short- and long-term toxicities and therapy should be continued for about 2 months after clinical remission. Major limitation of oral retinoids (acitretin) in children is the risk of growth retardation due to premature closure of epiphyses on long-term use. In an open-label study, three patients with psoriatic erythroderma were treated with etretinate in a dosage ranging from 0.5 to 0.9 mg/kg/d. After 4–5 months of treatment, they all had complete clearance of erythema and scaling. Etretinate was used as a treatment for plaque psoriasis in two children where both the patients had an excellent response.[29]

Cyclosporine is a noncytotoxic immunosuppressant that primarily acts by inhibiting T-cell function and thus, suppressing the interleukin (IL)-2 and interferon-γ and is effective in severe forms of psoriasis, such as pustular or erythrodermic psoriasis or when other therapies are ineffective. It is FDA approved for severe recalcitrant psoriasis in adults and for the prevention and treatment of transplant rejection in children older than 6 months. The studies involving the use of cyclosporine in pediatric psoriasis are very limited. Mahe et al.[30] reported unsatisfactory result in 4 patients, in whom cyclosporine was administered in a dose of 2.5–10 mg/kg. In an another review, three patients with pustular psoriasis have been described in whom the administered dose was from 1 to 2 mg/kg/day. Complete disappearance of lesions was seen in two patients who were treated for 12 and 6 months and the third patient showed a significant improvement after 5 months of treatment. The most commonly reported side effects with use of cyclosporine in pediatric age group include nausea, vomiting, diarrhoea, mild hypertension and changes in renal function.[31]

BIOLOGICAL AGENTS IN CHILDHOOD PSORIASIS

Biologics are drugs targeting cytokines like tumor necrosis factor that play an important role in the pathogenesis of psoriasis. These are an evolving therapeutic option for childhood psoriasis and since their action is targeted, so they lack many potential end-organ toxicities of traditional agents. However, there is a relative lack of long-term safety data in pediatric age group. Among all the available biologics, etanercept has been found to be overall effective and well tolerated in children and adolescents with moderate-to-severe plaque psoriasis. Etanercept is FDA approved for the treatment of adults with severe plaque psoriasis, psoriatic arthritis, rheumatoid arthritis and ankylosing spondylitis. In 2008, a double-blind, multicenter, phase 3, randomized controlled trial was conducted to evaluate the safety and efficacy of etanercept in pediatric psoriasis patients with moderate to severe plaque psoriasis. In this 48 week study, 211 ptients with psoriasis (4–17 years of age) were initially randomly assigned to a double-blind trial of 12 once-weekly subcutaneous injections of placebo or 0.8 mg of etanercept per kg of body weight (to a maximum of 50 mg), followed by 24 weeks of once-weekly open-label etanercept. At week 36, 138 patients underwent a second randomization to placebo or etanercept to investigate the effects of withdrawal and retreatment. The primary end point was 75% or greater improvement in PASI from baseline (PASI 75) at week 12. Adalimumab and infliximab have also been tried with variable results, but it is recommended that patients and families should be counselled about the possible increased risk of infections and malignancies in children.[32,33]

Thus, methotrexate, cyclosporine and TNF-α agonists can be used in the management of severe refractory pediatric psoriasis and hence, dermatologists should be aware of the use of these agents in difficult to treat cases of pediatric psoriasis. Since psoriasis as a chronic disease is punctuated by remissions and exacerbations and has a profound impact on the quality of life of the child, hence the family must learn to deal with the illness, considering the psychological burden on the child.

Points to Remember

- Psoriasis in children has few peculiar features which have been consistently observed in studies on childhood psoriasis. Guttate psoriasis is more common, spontaneous remissions are relatively more common than in adults while relapses usually follow infections. Certain clinical variants like erythroderma, localized and generalized pustular psoriasis and arthropathy are uncommon
- Western literature reports psoriasis prevalence to be around 0.71% in children
- Topical therapy remains the mainstay of treatment. Role of antibiotics remains controversial. Systemic therapies are used less often

REFERENCES

1. Beylot C, Puissant A, Bioulac P. Particular clinical features of psoriasis in infants and children. Acta Derma Venereol (Stockh). 1979;59(87):95-7.
2. Hutton KP, Orenberg EK, Jacobs AH. Childhood psoriasis. Cutis. 1987;39:26-7.
3. Manoharan R, Thomas J, Raneesha PK, Ragavi S, Manoharan D, Cynthia S. A study of childhood psoriasis. Indian J Paediatr Dermatol. 2013;14:23-5.
4. Dogra S, Kaur I. Childhood psoriasis. Indian J Dermatol Venereol Leprol. 2010;76:357-65.
5. Nanda A, Kaur S, Kaur I, Kumar B. Childhood psoriasis: An epidemiological survey of 112 patients. Pediatr Dermatol. 1990;7:19-21.
6. Morris A, Rogers M, Fischer G, Williams K. Childhood psoriasis: A clinical review of 1262 cases. Pediatr Dermatol. 2001;18:188-98.
7. Kumar B, Jain R, Sandhu K, Kumar B. Epidemiology of childhood psoriasis: A study of 419 patients from northern India. Int J Dermatol. 2004;43:654-8.
8. Benoit S, Hamm H. Childhood psoriasis. Clin Dermatol. 2007;25:555-62.
9. Dogra S, Kumar B. Epidemiology of skin diseases in school children: A study from Northern India. Pediatr Dermatol. 2003;20:470-3.
10. Sarkar R, Sharma RC, Koranne RV, Sardana K. Erythroderma in children: A clinico-etiological study. J Dermatol. 1999;26:507-11.
11. Nanda A, Kaur S, Kaur I, Kumar B. Childhood psoriasis: An epidemiological survey of 112 patients. Pediatr Dermatol. 1990;7:19-21.
12. Burden AD. Management of psoriasis in childhood. Clin Exp Dermatol. 1999;24:341-5.
13. Nyfors A. Psoriasis in children. Characteristics, prognosis and therapy: A review. Acta Derm Venereol (Stockh). 1981;95:47-53.
14. Fluhr JW, Cavallotti C, Berardesca E. Emollients, moisturizers, and keratolytic agents in psoriasis. Clin Dermatol. 2008;26:380-6.
15. Paghdal KV, Schwartz RA. Topical tar: Back to the future. J Am Acad Dermatol. 2009;61:294-302.
16. Lebwohl M, Ali S. Treatment of psoriasis. Part 1. Topical therapy and phototherapy. J Am Acad Dermatol. 2001;45:487-98.
17. Bhatia A, Mangat P, Jain B, Singh B, Katare OP. The developed lecithinized formulation, owing to its superior non-staining and washability characteristics, would potentially increase the acceptability of coal tar amongst patients. J Dermatolog Treat. 2008;19:105-10.
18. van de Kerkhof PC, Barker J, Griffiths CE, Kragballe K, Mason J, Menter A, et al. Psoriasis: Consensus on topical therapies. J Eur Acad Dermatol Venereol. 2008;22:859-70.
19. Cordoro KM. Topical therapy for the management of childhood psoriasis: Part I. Skin Therapy Lett. 2008; 13:1-3.
20. Travis LB, Silverberg NB. Psoriasis in infancy: Therapy with calcipotriene ointment. Cutis. 2001;68:341-4.
21. Diluvio L, Campione E, Paternç EJ, Mordenti C, El Hachem M, Chimenti S. Childhood nail psoriasis: A useful treatment with tazarotene 0.05%. Pediatr Dermatol. 2007;24:332-3.
22. Zvulunov A, Anisfeld A, Metzker A. Efficacy of short-contact therapy with dithranol in childhood psoriasis. Int J Dermatol. 1994;33:808-10.
23. Nyfors A. Psoriasis in children. Characteristics, prognosis and therapy: A review. Acta Derm Venereol (Stockh). 1981;95:47-53.
24. Brune A, Miller DW, Lin P, Cotrim-Russi D, Paller AS. Tacrolimus ointment is effective for psoriasis on the face and intertriginous areas in pediatric patients. Pediatr Dermatol. 2007;24:76-80.
25. Holme SA, Anstey AV. Phototherapy and PUVA photochemotherapy in children. Photodermatol Photoimmunol Photomed. 2004;20:69-75.
26. De Jager ME, de Jong EM, van de Kerkhof PC. Efficacy and safety of treatments for childhood psoriasis: A systematic literature review. J Am Acad Dermatol. 2010;62(6):1013-30.
27. Kumar B, Dhar S, Handa S. Methotrexate in childhood psoriasis. Paediatr Dermatol. 1994;11:271-73.
28. Warren RB, Chalmers RJ, Griffiths CE, Menter A. Methotrexate for psoriasis in the era of biological therapy. Clin Exp Dermatol. 2008;33:551-4.

29. Pang ML, Murase JE, Koo J. An updated review of acitretin-a systemic retinoid for the treatment of psoriasis. Expert Opin Drug Metab Toxicol. 2008;4:953-64.
30. Mahe E, Bodemer C, Pruszkowski A. Cyclosporine in childhood psoriasis. Arch Dermatol. 2001;137: 1532-33.
31. Perrett CM, Ilchyshyn A, Berth-Jones J. Cyclosporin in childhood psoriasis. J Dermatolog Treat. 2003;14:113-8.
32. Paller AS, Siegfried EC, Langley RG, Gottlieb AB, Pariser D, Landells I. Etanercept treatment for children and adolescents with plaque psoriasis. N Engl J Med. 2008;358:241-51.
33. Hawrot AC, Metry DW, Theos AJ. Etanercept for psoriasis in the paediatric population. Experience in nine patients. Paediatr Dermatol. 2006;23:67-71.

Chapter

17 Management of Psoriasis

Management of psoriasis is a challenge and broadly consists of topical therapy, systemic therapy, physical and complimentary therapies and biological therapy.

TOPICAL THERAPY

Psoriasis covering less than 5% of body surface area (BSA) can be managed in most patients with the use of topical agents alone. These agents are the cornerstone of treatment for most patients with psoriasis. Most patients with stable plaque psoriasis should be treated with topical therapy as it disturbs the patient's routine as little as possible. Tar preparations, vitamin D analogues, dithranol and corticosteroids are usually used for localized psoriasis.

Topical therapies, however, have the limitations that these cannot be used alone in extensive psoriasis and do not always work for nail psoriasis even though they are easy to administer and are readily available. In case of nail psoriasis, patients should be counseled to keep nails as short as possible, avoid manicures to prevent damage to the cuticles and prevent accumulation of any exogenous material under the nail. Any concomitant nail fungal infections should be treated appropriately.[1,2]

Various treatment modalities for psoriasis are given below:

Therapies used in the treatment of psoriasis

- Topical therapies: Emollients, keratolytics, corticosteroids, vitamin D analogues, omega 3 fatty acids, anthralin, coal tar and tazarotene
- Systemic Therapies: Methotrexate, cyclosporine, acitretin, oral vitamin D, phototherapy and photochemotherapy
- Various forms of phototherapy and photochemotherapy
- Biological agents: Anti-TNF agents (Infliximab, adalimumab, etanercept), T-cell targeted therapies (alefacept) and monoclonal antibody (ustekinumab)

Emollients

Emollients constitute the most important adjuvant therapy in the management of psoriasis. In mild psoriasis, emollient monotherapy may be sufficient. The various properties of emollients which are believed to help in psoriasis are as follows: Occlusive, humectant, antipruritic, anti-inflammatory, rehydrant and skin barrier restorant properties. In simple terms, they reduce water loss, prevent the skin from drying out and create a barrier against the environment. Emollients are particularly useful in inflammatory and chronic plaque psoriasis as well as in acral psoriasis. In psoriasis, emollients offer relief from dryness, scaling and cracking of the

TABLE 17.1: Various emollient agents and their properties

Emollients	Properties
Ceramides	Rehydrant
Glycerin	Humectant, rehydrant
Glycolic acid	Humectant
Lactic acid	Humectant, rehydrant
Lauromacrogol	Antipruritic
Paraffin, petroleum, oils	Occlusive, skin barrier restorant
Polyvinylpyrollidone	Skin barrier restorant
Salicylates	Anti-inflammatory, antioxidant and stabilizing agents
Urea	Humectant, rehydrant, keratolytic, penetration enhancing, epidermal thinning and antipruritic

skin and might also have an antiproliferative effect. Water-in-oil emollients have been shown to replace the requirement for daily use of other therapies in psoriasis.[3]

A number of emollients are used in psoriasis. Various emollient agents and their properties are given in Table 17.1.

Some authors recommend a daily warm bath followed by liberal application of emollients on wet skin together with one or two more moisturizing applications throughout the day. Full-body bath products that reduce scaling and improve stratum corneum hydration are of two types: dispersion bath oils and spreading bath oils. Similarly, in scalp psoriasis, a shampoo that encourages desquamation of the scalp should be used followed by the application of a keratolytic lotion.

The use of emollients is associated with side effects, such as irritant dermatitis, allergic contact dermatitis, stinging, cosmetic acne and pigmentation disorders.

Keratolytics

Keratolytics form the cornerstone of therapy for psoriasis. There are a number of keratolytic agents available for the treatment of psoriasis and the most widely used and oldest keratolytic agent known today, salicylic acid is available in concentrations ranging from 0.5% to 60% in a number of vehicles. It is particularly useful in thick scaly plaque psoriasis. Salicylic acid can be used as monotherapy in some patients. It can also be added to anthralin and zinc pastes to reduce the interaction between these two ingredients. Additionally, salicylic acid offers antioxidant properties to such preparations.

Application on large areas and in concentrations greater than 10% results in toxicity (salicylism). It is seen especially in children and manifests as oral mucosal burning, frontal headache, central nervous system symptoms, metabolic acidosis, tinnitus, nausea, vomiting, and gastric symptoms. Salicylic acid may reduce the action of other therapies for psoriasis, including calcipotriene.

Urea has both emollient and keratolytic properties. Furthermore, it can be combined with anthralin to improve its clinical efficacy. Urea combined with bifonazole is useful in the management of scalp psoriasis. It is used topically in concentrations of 5% to 25% in creams or lotions and up to 40% in nail preparations.[4]

Omega Fatty Acids

Abnormal serum fatty acid profile has been noted in psoriasis. Emollients and moisturisers containing omega fatty acids (omega 3 and omega 6 fatty acid preparations) have been found to help in the restoration of skin barrier in psoriasis. Olive oil has been particularly useful in this respect.[5]

Corticosteroids

Among all the available treatment modalities for psoriasis, corticosteroids are the most widely used. In USA, they are the mainstay of topical treatment. In appropriate concentrations, they are the treatment of choice on the face and neck, flexures and genitalia. Corticosteroids have the merits of ease of application and removal, lack of irritancy and the absence of staining of skin or linen. Various corticosteroids vary in their potency. The potency of earlier corticosteroids has been enhanced by chemical modification including halogenation, acetylation and methylation. The penetration of corticosteroids can be enhanced by using occlusive dressings or changing the base they are formulated in. Potent and very potent steroids are more useful than mild-to-moderate steroids in psoriasis. The corticosteroids have the disadvantage that these cannot be used for longer periods of time. The hazards of corticosteroid therapy are now well known, and are especially increased by using occlusive dressings. Long-term effects include skin atrophy, telangiectasia, striae, purpura, iatrogenic Cushing's syndrome and hypothalamic-pituitary-adrenal (HPA) axis suppression. The regimens to minimize the long-term effects are yet to be recognized. The effects of tachyphylaxis are not well documented due to the lack of long-term studies.

On the scalp and other parts of the body, corticosteroids can be tried if tar has failed and dithranol is inappropriate or unsuccessful. Shampoos and foams containing clobetasol propionate have shown improvement in 2 weeks in scalp psoriasis. Potent topical corticosteroids may be useful in subungual hyperkeratosis, especially in combination with salicylic acid, as well as in pitting and ridging. However, long-term use may result in skin and even phalanx atrophy.

Intralesional corticosteroids, particularly triamcinolone, are administered via a 28-gauge needle and syringe or a 29-gauge insulin syringe. These agents are particularly useful in pitting, ridging, nail thickening and subungual hyperkeratosis. In addition to pain, patients may experience periungual hypopigmentation, subungual hemorrhage, and reversible atrophy.[6]

Indications of topical corticosteroids are:

- Mild-to-moderate psoriasis (BSA<10%)
- Severe psoriasis(BSA>10%), in combination with other topical agents, such as anthralin, tar or vitamin D3 analogues
- Scalp psoriasis
- Flexural and facial psoriasis (although calcineurin inhibitors are preferred).

Contraindications of topical steroids are:

- Any active infection
- Involvement of face, flexures, eyelids and genitalia
- Allergic contact dermatitis to corticosteroids or the vehicle base.

VITAMIN D ANALOGUES

Calcitriol, the naturally occurring metabolite of vitamin D and its three synthetic analogues calcipotriol, tacalcitol and maxacalcitol (1,25-dihydroxyvitamin D_3) have all been shown to be effective topical treatment for mild psoriasis. These analogues (i.e. calcitriol, calcipotriene, tacalcitol and maxacalcitol) affect cellular differentiation and proliferation via vitamin D receptor mediated effects on the proliferation and differentiation of epidermal keratinocytes and on the immunological features of psoriasis, including shifting the Th1 cytokine profile of plaques towards a Th2 cytokine profile. Additionally, they regulate apoptosis and demonstrate an immunomodulatory effect. All vitamin D analogues allow a reduction in the duration and potency of other treatments. They are odorless and nonstaining and therefore, cosmetically more acceptable than anthralin.

Calcitriol is an active and naturally occurring metabolite of vitamin D_3, 1,25-dihydroxy-vitamin D_3. Calcipotriol, tacalcitol and maxacalcitol are three synthetic analogues of vitamin D_3. All three cause hypercalcemia but are safe if used according to their respective dosage regimens. Other side effects include pruritus, burning, edema, peeling, dryness and erythema which diminish with ongoing treatment. A model vitamin D analogue that has minor calcemic activity is yet to be developed. Calcipotriene (also known as calcipotriol internationally) is slightly more effective than calcitriol and tacalcitol and is as effective and potent (but not ultrapotent) as topical corticosteroids. A combination of calcipotriene with betamethasone reduces the long-term side effects of each ingredient by 1 year. Furthermore, since the combination has a low systemic absorption, the localized anti-inflammatory and immunoregulatory effect is higher than that of either of the individual drugs used separately. The combination is also available as a topical solution that is useful in the management of scalp psoriasis, with better efficacy and less irritation. In subungual hyperkeratosis (nail psoriasis), calcipotriene may be used alone or in combination with corticosteroids.

The concentration of calcipotriene used is 0.005%, and it should not be applied more than twice daily. The upper limit per week is 100 g of cream or ointment or 60 mL of scalp solution in adults. If both cream and scalp solution are used, the limit per week is either 60 g of cream and 30 mL of solution or 30 g of cream and 60 mL of solution. In children, the maximum dose is 50 g for those aged 6 to 12 years and 75 g for children above 12 years per week.

About 10% of patients using calcipotriene may notice a mild dermatitis as a side effect, when used on easily irritated areas such as face, hairline and flexural areas (hence calcitriol is preferred at these sites). Calcipotriene also has a limited effect on calcium homeostasis as compared to calcitriol and tacalcitol.

Compliance is better with tacalcitol since it only needs to be used once daily as opposed to the others, which are used twice daily. In addition to the side effects associated with calcitriol, it can also cause paresthesias. Tacalcitol is not available in the US.[7]

Indications of topical vitamin D3 analogues:

- Mild-to-moderate psoriasis (BSA<10%). As monotherapy or in combination with other agents such as topical corticosteroids
- Severe psoriasis (BSA>10%). Here caution should be exercised to avoid hypercalcemia
- Scalp psoriasis and nail psoriasis. Good results have been reported in various studies.

Contraindications of topical vitamin D3 analogues:

- Erythroderma and severe psoriasis, with BSA involvement requiring more than 100g/week of calcipotriol/calcipotriene
- Allergy to vitamin D3 analogues or vehicle/base of the constituents
- Sarcoidosis and other conditions characterized by hypercalcemia such as bone metastases
- Renal insufficiency.

Tazarotene

Tazarotene is a synthetic retinoid, whose main metabolite, tazarotenic acid binds to RARs β and γ. This is a topical vitamin A derivative that is modified to tazarotenic acid through de-esterification in the skin. It appears to exert its beneficial effects in psoriasis by modulating cell proliferation and differentiation. Tazarotene can only be used once daily, and therefore has limited use as monotherapy. It is less potent than vitamin D analogues and moderate or potent local corticosteroids. Tazarotene is used in patients in whom over 20% of the body surface area (BSA) is affected. It is available in a 0.05% or 0.1% gel. The starting dose is a 0.05% gel that can be increased to 0.1% as needed. It is normally used for 12 weeks at a time. The main drawback of tazarotene is local irritation at the site of application. The use of tazarotene for psoriasis may exacerbate acne. Since tazarotene is teratogenic, it should not be used by individuals who are pregnant or planning a pregnancy.[8]

Indications of topical tazarotene in psoriasis are:

- Mild-to-moderate psoriasis, as monotherapy or in combination
- Palmoplantar psoriasis.

Contraindications to the use of tazarotene in psoriasis are:

- Erythrodermic psoriasis
- Pregnancy and lactation
- Unstable psoriasis
- Allergic contact dermatitis to tazarotene or any of the constituents of the formulation.

Anthralin

Dithranol or anthralin (1,8-dihydroxy-9-anthrone) is a synthetic derivative of chrysarobin, a tree-bark extract. This drug has been used in the treatment of psoriasis for over 80 years, but due to its staining properties, it is not a cosmetically acceptable agent. Various studies have demonstrated that it posesses lower efficacy than topical corticosteroids and vitamin D derivatives as monotherapy. Salicylic acid is added to stabilize the dithranol formulations. It is thought to exert its effects through its action on mitochondria. Currently, anthralin is used for the management of subacute and chronic psoriasis in two ways—conventional and short-contact treatment.

Conventional treatment is initiated with 0.1% anthralin ointment or paste that is applied to the lesions only for 30 minutes to few hours and then washed-off. If irritation occurs, the strength and contact time must be reduced. The strength is gradually increased to 0.5% and even up to 1%, and the contact period is extended to overnight. Short-contact treatment involves applying anthralin to the lesion in strengths of 0.1% to 2% for up to 60 minutes daily and then washing it off.

Treatment should be continued until the psoriasis clears. Since anthralin causes skin irritation and staining of the skin, clothing and furniture, it is best used less often. In many cases it is combined with coal tar to reduce irritation. Furthermore, it can be combined with phototherapy for better results.

Anthralin ointment applied on nails and washed-off after 30 minutes is useful in onycholysis and subungual hyperkeratosis. However, this treatment results in temporary staining of the nail and local irritation.

Precautions to be taken while using anthralin:

- The use of anthralin should be avoided on the face, skin flexures and genitals
- Hands should be washed thoroughly after use
- Anthralin should not be used in acute/unstable psoriasis, pustular psoriasis or applied onto inflamed skin
- It is useful to inform patients that staining slowly disappears upon discontinuation of treatment.[9]

Indications of anthralin in psoriasis are:

Mild-to-moderate or severe psoriasis as monotherapy or in combination with other treatment modalities such as phototherapy.

Contraindications to the use of anthralin in psoriasis are:

- Erythroderma
- Generalized/localized pustular psoriasis
- Unstable psoriasis.

Coal Tar

Coal tar is a complex mixture of thousands of substances produced by primary condensation during the carbonization of coal. Tar has been used in the topical therapy of psoriasis for more than a century. It is believed to have an antimitotic effect but this is not proven. Its use in psoriasis was popularised by Goeckerman, and, for more than a century, his regimen of daily application of 2–5% crude coal tar, combined with a tar bath and UV-light, has been a mainstay of in-patient treatment. Coal tar reduces the thickness of the epidermis and has a slightly antipruritic and antiseptic effect. It is particularly useful in the management of stable chronic plaque psoriasis. Coal tar is a mixture of thousands of compounds and is available as crude coal tar, solutions, ointments, as well as shampoos that can be used for scalp psoriasis. The crude form is less acceptable cosmetically (due to its unpleasant odor and staining properties), but is more effective than the purified preparations.

Coal tar therapy is initiated with concentrations of 0.5% to 1% of crude coal tar and increased every few days up to 10%. Broad band or narrow band phototherapy is usually used to enhance the effect of coal tar therapy, with coal tar being applied about 2 hours before the light exposure. The Ingram regimen includes the application of anthralin following coal tar and light therapy.

Side-effects of Coal Tar

Coal tar causes skin irritation, folliculitis, unpleasant odor and staining of clothing and is quite messy to use. Coal tar has a carcinogenic potential, and gloves should be worn by anyone handling it, including individuals making coal tar preparations.[10]

Goeckerman therapy for psoriasis was first described at the Mayo Clinic in 1925 by American dermatologist William H Goeckerman and continues to be used due to its safety and efficacy, although various modifications have been made to the original regimen. The standard therapy includes the use of 2–5% crude coal tar in a petrolatum base applied daily to the psoriatic plaques. The minimum period of time of tar application is 2 hours, although greater periods of time produce better results. The patient is then exposed to broad-band/ narrow-band ultraviolet light.

Ingram regimen involves the use of a tar bath in which scales and the previous applications are removed, followed by suberythema UVB and then the lesions are precisely covered with dithranol paste. The initial concentration is 0.05% or 0.1%, increasing cautiously up to 4% according to response and aiming to avoid irritation of the normal or psoriatic skin. The paste is kept in position with tubular gauze or stockingette. After 18–22 hours, the cycle is repeated and can be on an in-patient or day-care basis.

Points to Remember

- Management of psoriasis is a challenge and broadly consists of topical therapy, systemic therapy, physical and complimentary therapies and biological therapy
- Psoriasis covering less than 5% of BSA can be managed in most patients with the use of topical agents alone. These agents are the cornerstone of treatment for most patients with psoriasis
- Goeckerman therapy for psoriasis was first described at the Mayo Clinic in 1925 and is offered in various day care clinics

REFERENCES

1. Menter A, Korman NJ, Elmets CA, Feldman SR, Gelfand JM, Gordon KB, et al. Guidelines of care for the management of psoriasis and psoriatic arthritis: section 4. Guidelines of care for the management and treatment of psoriasis with traditional systemic agents. J Am Acad Dermatol. 2009;61(3):451-85.
2. Mason AR, Mason J, Cork M, Dooley G, Edwards G. Topical treatments for chronic plaque psoriasis. Cochrane Database Syst Rev. 2009;CD005028.
3. Feldman SR. Tachyphylaxis to topical corticosteroids: the more you use them, the less they work? Clin Dermatol 2006;24(3):229–30.
4. Fluhr JW, Cavallotti C, Berardesca E. Emollients, moisturizers, and keratolytic agents in psoriasis. Clin Dermatol 2008;26:380-6.
5. Mayser P, Mrowietz U, Arenberger P, Bartak P, Buchvald J, Christophers E, et al. Omega-3 fatty acid-based lipid infusion in patients with chronic plaque psoriasis: results of a double-blind, randomized, placebo-controlled, multicenter trial. J Am Acad Dermatol. 1998;38(4):539-47.
6. Kaplan DH, Barker J. Psoriasis. N Engl J Med 2009;361:496-509.

7. Rim JH, Choe YB, Youn JI. Positive effect of using calcipotriol ointment with narrow-band ultraviolet B phototherapy in psoriatic patients. Photodermatol Photoimmunol Photomed 2002;18:131-4.
8. Diluvio L, Campione E, Paternç EJ, Mordenti C, El Hachem M, Chimenti S. Childhood nail psoriasis: A useful treatment with tazarotene 0.05%. Pediatr Dermatol 2007;24:332-3.
9. Zvulunov A, Anisfeld A, Metzker A. Efficacy of short-contact therapy with dithranol in childhood psoriasis. Int J Dermatol 1994;33(11):808-10.
10. Paghdal KV, Schwartz RA. Topical tar: back to the future. J Am Acad Dermatol 2009;61:294-302. w

Chapter

18 Systemic Therapies for Psoriasis

Psoriasis is a chronic immune mediated cutaneous disorder that can significantly affect patient's quality of life (QoL). Although the exact etiopathogenesis remains to be elucidated, immunologic abnormalities with an increase in immune mediators are likely primary contributing factors. Most patients have mild disease that can be adequately managed by topical therapy. However, a subset of the psoriatic patient's with severe disease requires phototherapy and/or systemic treatment. Due to its chronic and recalcitrant course, a combinational approach (including topical, systemic and nondrug interventions) is often necessary for successful long-term management.

Of the conventional systemic agents, acitretin, cyclosporine and methotrexate are the most commonly used. In the new era of biologics, these agents remain as valuable therapeutic options for severe psoriasis. Recent studies have also provided insights into enhanced efficacy and safety when these drugs are used in combination with the biologics. However, because systemic treatment carries a higher risk for adverse effects, moderate to severe cases are best managed under the supervision of dermatologists, who are more familiar with the use of these agents.[1]

TREATMENT RATIONALE

The appropriate management of psoriasis depends on several factors, including findings from diagnostic investigations, extent and severity of psoriasis, treatment history, age and patient preferences. Besides achieving tangible clinical improvements, the adopted therapeutic approach must also minimize the quality of life (QoL) impairment, such as discomfort, disability and heighten self-consciousness, which can lead to social avoidance behaviors. Consequently, early diagnosis and ongoing medical and adjunctive care are crucial for controlling chronicity and disease severity.[2]

Biologics represent the newest class of antipsoriatic agents, although their advent has revolutionized the treatment of moderate to severe psoriasis, long-term safety remains to be established and their high cost can be prohibitive. The most commonly used traditional systemic agents (i.e. acitretin, cyclosporine and methotrexate) continue to have a place in the management of severe psoriasis and novel combined uses have emerged.[3]

REFERENCES

1. Ingram JT. The approach to psoriasis. BMJ 1953;II:591-4.
2. Gaikwad R, Deshpande S, Raje S, Dhamdhere DV, Ghate MR. Evaluation of functional impairment in psoriasis. Indian J Dermatol Venereol Leprol 2006;72:37-40.
3. Ameen M, Smith HR, Barker JNWN. Combined mycophenolate mofetil and ciclosporin therapy for severe recalcitrant psoriasis. Clin Exp Dermatol. 2001;26:480-3.

Chapter 19

Retinoids in Psoriasis

The term retinoids has been applied to a family of natural and synthetic analogues of vitamin A. Retinoids are vitamin A derivatives, which modulate epidermal proliferation and differentiation, have immunomodulatory as well as anti-inflammatory properties. Etretinate, acitretin and isotretinoin are the retinoids which have been used in psoriasis for many decades now. Etretinate is little used nowadays as it has been superseded in many countries by acitretin, which has a shorter half-life. Acitretin, the active metabolite of etretinate, is the most commonly used oral retinoid for psoriasis. It is less effective compared to methotrexate and cyclosporine as monotherapy and requires 3–6 months to achieve maximal response. It has been used in different doses in clinical trials and the results are largely dose dependent.[1]

Acitretin as monotherapy is particularly considered to be effective in exfoliative erythrodermic psoriasis and pustular psoriasis. It has been extensively used in combination with ultraviolet B (UVB) or PUVA therapy for chronic plaque type psoriasis with enhanced efficacy, reduced treatment frequency, duration, and cumulative UV doses, resulting in a more effective, convenient and safer treatment.

The important advantages with this drug are chemoprevention against malignancy and that it is not immunosuppressive. Therefore, it is the drug of choice in human immunodeficiency virus (HIV) positive patients with psoriasis and is also used as combination therapy with biologics.

Acitretin has significant adverse effects like teratogenic potential, hyperlipidemia, mucocutaneous side effects, diffuse idiopathic hyperostosis, liver toxicity, and pseudotumor cerebri-like symptoms. Women of childbearing age should use adequate contraception for at least 3 years after discontinuing the use of acitretin. Isotretinoin is an option in women of childbearing age as its elimination half-life is short and adequate contraception should be maintained for at least 1 month after stopping the drug.[2,3]

Newer generation retinoids (tazarotene) are increasingly being used for psoriasis because of their better pharmacokinetic properties and selectivity for the beta and gamma subtypes of retinoic acid receptors (RARs), resulting in targeted action on psoriatic keratinocytes, thereby minimizing the risk of adverse effects. The wash out period of tazarotene is short due to shorter half-life of 7–12 hours of its active metabolite, tazarotenic acid. Therefore, the contraception may only be necessary for a few days after the last dose. Tazarotene has been found to be an effective, safer and better tolerated oral retinoid for psoriasis patients in phase III studies. This drug has been safely used for up to 52 weeks. Unlike other retinoids, it does not significantly increase the prevalence of hypertriglyceridemia, hypercholesterolemia, abnormal liver function test results, scaling, eye dryness, or alopecia.[4]

Bexarotene is a synthetic retinoid X receptor (RXR)—selective retinoid. In a phase II multicentric study, >50% improvement in modified PASI, plaque elevation and physician's global assessment was seen in 22, 52 and 36% of patients, respectively.[5]

Retinoids have several advantages over conventional systemic drugs like they are not immunosuppressive, there is no limitation of cumulative dose, and they cause no significant hepatic or renal toxicity. Therefore, these are good candidates for combination and maintenance therapy both with conventional systemic antipsoriatic drugs as well as with the biologic agents.[6]

ACITRETIN[7-11]

Pregnancy category—X

Acitretin is the main active metabolite of etretinate (an ester). Acitretin has the great advantage of less half-life than etretinate due to decreased lipophilicity since it is a free acid. Acitretin is a second generation aromatic retinoid (a vitamin A derivative). Acitretin is indicated mainly for men and for postmenopausal women. Due to its teratogenic potential, premenopausal women are generally excluded as treatment candidates. Acitretin is the safest oral systemic agent for psoriasis, apart from its teratogenic risk that persists 2–3 years following treatment discontinuation. The mechanism of action of acitretin includes inhibiting cell replication by controlling cellular differentiation within the epidermis. It has been found to decrease inflammation as well.

Advantages and Benefits of Acitretin

- Acitretin is the safest oral systemic agent for psoriasis, apart from its teratogenic risk that persists 2–3 years following treatment discontinuation
- Convenient once daily oral dosing
- Acitretin is very helpful as an adjunct to phototherapy
- Acitretin is highly effective for treating pustular (including palmoplantar psoriasis) or erythrodermic forms of psoriasis. However, it is less effective as monotherapy for plaque psoriasis
- Acitretin usually does not cause organ damage, which is a side-effect with other drugs (such as methotrexate and cyclosporine), therefore, it can be used for long-term maintenance therapy
- No risk of immunosuppression. Hence, it is used in psoriatic patients with HIV and for psoriasis patients with a history of melanoma, acitretin should be considered as a therapeutic option.

Risks and Side-effects of Acitretin

- Therapeutic response is usually seen in 2–4 months. The main issue with compliance is to minimize side-effects through inclusion of topical agents and phototherapy
- It can usually be used in combination with phototherapy or biological agents

- The most common side-effects noted with the use of acitretin include dryness and irritation of the skin, lips, eyes, nose and mucous membranes. Thus, frequent use of a moisturizer is recommended to reduce the irritation. Due to the medication's drying effects, starting with a lower dose may ease the intensity. Other adverse side-effects include elevation of cholesterol and triglyceride levels, liver toxicity, bone changes and alopecia.
- Due to the serious risk of teratogenecity, acceptable methods of birth control must be practiced by and discussed with the patient. Because of its relatively long bioelimination, even following treatment cessation, female patients must continue to avoid pregnancy for the next 2–3 years.

Recommendations for Acitretin

Indications of acitretin in psoriasis are:

- Erythrodermic psoriasis
- Pustular psoriasis
- Severe psoriasis that cannot be managed with topical treatments or phototherapy or photochemotherapy
- In combination with other treatment modalities such as phototherapy for chronic plaque psoriasis.

Acitretin is FDA approved for adults with severe plaque type psoriasis; 0.5–1 mg/kg/day is given as a single dose. Lower doses (≤25 mg/d) are often used to minimize side effects, especially in combination regimens. When acitretin is added to UV light, light dose should be reduced by 30%–50%.

Efficacy rates are not well-defined but are high, based on the studies of high dosages that are poorly tolerated. Efficacy rates when used in combination with phototherapy are higher.

Long-term Results: Not reported.

Contraindications of acitretin in psoriasis are:

- Acitretin is a potent teratogen and must be avoided in women of childbearing potential
- Severely impaired liver or kidney function
- Chronic abnormally elevated blood lipid values
- Concomitant hepatotoxic drug such as methotrexate intake
- Pancreatitis, excessive alcohol intake
- Poorly controlled diabetes mellitus
- Hypertriglyceridemia
- Pregnancy and lactation.

Mothers receiving acitretin should not breastfeed. The safety and efficacy of acitretin in children with psoriasis is not established; high-dose, long-term oral retinoid use has been associated with ossification of interosseous ligaments and tendons of the extremities, skeletal hyperostosis, decrease in bone mineral density, and premature epiphyseal closure.

TOXICITY

Presence of following features is an indication of the toxicity/overdosage: Cheilitis, alopecia, xerosis, pruritus, xerophthalmia, night blindness, dry mouth, paronychia, paresthesias, headache, pseudotumor cerebri, nausea, abdominal pain, arthralgias, myalgias, hypertriglyceridemia and abnormal liver function test (LFT) results.

Drug Interactions

- Etretinate can be formed with concurrent ingestion of acitretin and ethanol
- Acitretin may potentiate glucose-lowering effect of glibenclamide
- Acitretin may interfere with the contraceptive effect of microdosed progestin minipill180
- Acitretin and methotrexate can both cause hepatotoxicity; therefore, they should be combined with caution
- Acitretin may reduce the protein binding of phenytoin
- Acitretin and tetracyclines can both increase intracranial pressure; their combined use should be avoided (pseudotumor cerebri)
- Concomitant administration of vitamin A and other oral retinoids with acitretin should be avoided.

Preacitretin screening/Baseline monitoring should include:
- History and physical examination to exclude contraindications
- CBC, LFT, KFT, blood sugar and lipid profile
- Consider spinal X-ray(often initially performed during the first 3 months of therapy if long-term treatment is anticipated).

Evaluation during acitretin treatment.
- LFT, lipid profile should be repeated at 2-week intervals for the first 8 weeks, then every 6–12 weeks
- CBC and renal function tests every 3 months
- Pregnancy test if indicated
- Monitor mucocutaneous side effects
- Monitor for the development of hyperostosis by X-ray of spine (once yearly in patients receiving long-term treatment).

Pregnancy: Category X.

Psoriatic Arthritis: Generally thought to be ineffective for psoriatic arthritis.

Points to Remember

- Acitretin, the active metabolite of etretinate, is the most commonly used oral retinoid for psoriasis
- Acitretin as monotherapy is particularly considered to be effective in exfoliative erythrodermic psoriasis and pustular psoriasis. It has been extensively used in combination with ultraviolet B (UVB) or PUVA therapy for chronic plaque type psoriasis
- Retinoids have several advantages over conventional systemic drugs like they are not immunosuppressive, there is no limitation of cumulative dose and they cause no significant hepatic or renal toxicity. Therefore, these are good candidates for combination and maintenance therapy both with conventional systemic antipsoriatic drugs as well as with the biologic agents

REFERENCES

1. Lowe NJ, Lzarus V, Matt L. Systemic retinoids for psoriasis. J Am Acad Dermatol. 1988;19:186-91.
2. Murray HE, Anhalt AW, Lessard R, Schacter RK, Ross JB, Stewart WD, A. 12 month treatment of severe psoriasis with acitretin: results of a Canadian open multicenter study. J Am Acad Dermatol. 1991;24(4):598-602.
3. Kragballe K, Jansen C, Geiger JM, et al. A double-blind comparison of acitretin and etretinate in the treatment of severe psoriasis. Results of a Nordic multicentre study. Acta Derm Venereol. 1989;69(1):35-40.
4. Gollnick HPM. Oral retinoids: efficacy and toxicity in psoriasis. Br J Dermatol. 1996;135(49):6-17.
5. Bollag W. Chemistry and pharmacology of retinoids. In: Farber EM, Cox AJ. (Eds). Psoriasis. Proceedings of the third international symposium. New York: Grune & Stratton.1982:pp.175-83.
6. Orfanos CE, Steigleder GK, Pullmann H, et al. Oral retinoid and UVB radiation. Acta Derm Venereol. 1979;59:241-4.
7. Gollnick H, Zaun H, Ruzicka T, et al. Relapse rate of severe generalized psoriasis after treatment with acitretin or etretinate. Results the first randomized double-blind multicenter half-year follow-up study. Eur J Dermatol. 1993;3:442-6.
8. Van Dooren-Greebe R, Lemmens JA, De Boo T, Hangx NM, Kuijpers AL, Van de Kerkhof PC. Prolonged treatment with oral retinoids in adults: no influence on the frequency and severity of spinal abnormalities. Br J Dermatol. 1996;134(1):71-6.
9. Brindley CJ. Overview of recent clinical pharmacokinetic studies with acitretin (Ro 10-1670, etretin). Dermatologica. 1989;178(2):79-87.
10. Gronhoj-Larsen F, Steinkjer B, Jakobsen P, Hjorter A, Brockhoff PB, Nielsen-Kudsk F. Acitretin is converted to etretinate only during concomitant alcohol intake. Br J Dermatol. 2000;143(6):1164-9.
11. Roenigk HH Jr, Callen JP, Guzzo CA, et al. Effects of acitretin on the liver. J Am Acad Dermatol. 1999;41:584-8.

Chapter

20

Calcineurin Inhibitors in Psoriasis

Cyclosporine is a cyclic undecapeptide derived from the fungus *Tolypocladium inflatum* Gams. Cyclosporine (CSA) has the highest efficacy among all the nonbiologic systemic therapies. It is called the crisis drug as it is effective in cases resistant to other modalities and brings rapid control even in very severe cases. The ability of cyclosporine to clear skin lesions of psoriasis was first noted in four patients in 1979, as an incidental finding during a trial of this drug in inflammatory arthritis. The mechanism of action of cyclosporine in psoriasis is not entirely known, but it is believed to act via its inhibitory effects on T-cell activation. Cyclosporine (CSA) is given in doses of 2.5–5 mg/kg/day. Many studies have shown that CSA, when used for 12–16 weeks, leads to a significant improvement in psoriasis in up to 80–90% of patients. This drug has been found to be useful in the management of childhood psoriasis also. A recent review of its use in children has suggested that the side-effect profile is similar to that of adults. The main problems with CSA are drug-induced hypertension, renal side-effects, increased incidence of malignancy and rebound flare after stopping the drug. Long-term therapy results in permanent renal scarring and loss of function. Patients who are treated with CSA for more than 2 years continuously have especially high risk of developing irreversible renal damage. To avoid this dreaded complication, CSA should be given in intermittent courses of maximum 12 weeks duration. Another concern with CSA is the increased incidence of cutaneous squamous cell carcinomas (SCC), especially in patients who have previously received PUVA (psoralen + UV A) therapy. In a large (5-year follow up) cohort study, evaluating more than 1200 subjects on long-term CSA, there was a sixfold increased risk of nonmelanoma skin cancers, especially SCC, in patients who had received additional PUVA therapy, whereas the incidence of internal malignancy was not found to be high as compared to the general population.[1,2]

Tacrolimus, a calcineurin inhibitor has been tested in severe recalcitrant psoriasis patients with good response, after an initial observation of the improvement of psoriasis in one heart and three liver transplant patients who had recieved tacrolimus. Subsequently, a double-blind, placebo-controlled study conducted by European FK 506 multicenter psoriasis study group reported 83% PASI reduction in 27 psoriasis patients at the end of 9 weeks.[3]

Pimecrolimus and voclosporine, are newer calcineurin inhibitors which are believed to possess higher efficacy and better side-effect profile, and are increasingly being tried in psoriasis. Oral pimecrolimus was initially used by Rappersberger et al. with high clinical efficacy and good tolerability. Subsequently, in a large, double-blind clinical trial, pimecrolimus was given in doses of 20 and 30 mg twice daily in psoriasis patients. A mean percentage reduction in PASI of 51.3% and 54% at week 7 from the baseline was observed in 20 and 30 mg group, respectively. The drug was noted to be well tolerated and there were no clinically relevant abnormalities in the laboratory parameters.[4]

Voclosporine is a novel calcineurin inhibitor having higher affinity for calcineurin and faster clearance of its metabolites from the body, as compared to cyclosporine. Voclosporine with high efficacy comparable to cyclosporine and better safety profile is a promising future therapy for psoriasis. The drug has been found to be effective in psoriasis in phase II and III studies. In phase II studies, PASI 75 response was achieved in 67% of cases receiving 1.5 mg/kg/day of voclosporine without any significant side-effects. In a phase III clinical trial, 451 plaque psoriasis patients received either voclosporine (in a dose of 0.2, 0.3 and 0.4 mg/kg) or placebo. At the end of 12 weeks, PASI 75 response was achieved in the voclosporine 0.2, 0.3 and 0.4 mg/kg groups by 16, 25 and 47% of patients, respectively, and in the placebo group by only 4% of patients.[5]

CYCLOSPORINE[6-11]

Strength of recommendation—B
Level of evidence—II
Pregnancy category status—Category C

Cyclosporine is an immunosuppressant that is frequently used in organ transplantation. Although cyclosporine is a very effective antipsoriatic agent, it is generally reserved for patients with severe disabling, or recalcitrant psoriasis (also referred to as a crisis drug), owing to its cost and potentially serious side-effect profile (e.g. renal impairment). Cyclosporine offers rapid disease control in severe cases by suppressing the body's immune system and slowing the rapid production of skin cells.

Advantages and Benefits of cyclosporine

- It is administered orally 1–2 times daily
- The onset of effect is rapid (4–8 weeks); improvement is often seen within the first 4 weeks
- It is highly effective for severe psoriasis, especially helpful for treating acute flare-ups
- It can be used intermittently in short-term courses or combined with other topical and systemic therapies
- Multiple short courses are recommended to reduce the potential for toxicity.

Risks and Side-effects of Cyclosporine

- The long-term use of cyclosporine leads to kidney damage, although the damage is often reversible with treatment cessation
- The total duration of therapy should not exceed 1–2 years to avoid severe adverse systemic effects
- Regular assessments through blood and urine tests, and blood pressure monitoring are required throughout treatment
- Rebounds are common if the drug is tapered rapidly or when the medication is stopped
- Side-effects include flu-like symptoms, nausea, diarrhea, hair growth, high blood pressure, numbness and tingling, and kidney damage

- Because cyclosporine suppresses the body's immune system, there is an increased risk of infections and certain cancers, such as skin cancer and lymphomas, but reported incidences usually involve use in organ transplantation where the medication is administered long-term and at higher doses
- Cyclosprine cannot be used at the same time with psoralen + UVA (PUVA) or UVB phototherapy, methotrexate or other immunosuppressive agents, coal tar, or radiation therapy
- As a potent immunosuppressive agent, increasing the risk of skin cancer, patients being treated with cyclosporine should be advised to take sun-protective measures (viz; applying a broad-spectrum sunscreen daily and wearing long-sleeved clothing and hats).

Indications of Cyclosporine

- Erythrodermic psoriasis
- Generalized pustular psoriasis and palmoplantar psoriasis
- Adult, nonimmunocompromised patients with severe, recalcitrant psoriasis
- Some guidelines suggest the use of cyclosporine in moderate to severe psoriasis.

Note

- ❖ Severe is defined by the US Food and Drug Administration (FDA) as extensive or disabling plaque psoriasis
- ❖ Recalcitrant is defined by the FDA as those patients who have failed to respond to at least one systemic therapy or in patients for whom other systemic therapies are contraindicated, or cannot be tolerated.

Dosing

The recommended dose of cyclosporine in psoriasis is 2.5–5.0 mg/kg/day in two divided doses/day. The dose should be decreased by 0.5–1.0 mg/kg when clearance is achieved or when hypertension or decreased renal function test results are observed.

Duration of Dosing

It is optimally used as interventional therapy (3–4 months) and may be repeated at intervals after a resting period.

US approval: One year continuous treatment
Non-US approval: 2 years continuous treatment.

Evidence of efficacy: Many studies have shown that cyclosporine (CSA), when used for 12–16 weeks, leads to a significant improvement in psoriasis in up to 80–90% of patients. This drug has been found to be useful in the management of childhood psoriasis also. At 3 and 5 mg/kg/day, 36% and 65%, respectively, achieve a clear or almost clear result after 8 weeks. After 8–16 weeks, 50–70% of patients achieve PASI 75. The long-term use is not recommended because of toxicities and the disadvantage of rapid relapse after abrupt discontinuation of cyclosporine.

Transplant recipients as young as 1 year have been treated with no unusual adverse events; although safety and efficacy of cyclosporine for children <18 years with psoriasis have not been established, it may be considered in this patient population with severe psoriasis.

Contraindications

The contraindications to the use of cyclosporine are:

- Impaired renal function
- Uncontrolled hypertension
- Concomitant psoralen plus ultraviolet A (PUVA) or ultraviolet B (UVB), methotrexate or other immunosuppressive agents, coal tar, history of >200 PUVA treatments or radiation therapy
- Malignancy
- Primary or secondary immunodeficiency
- Concomitant immunosuppressive therapy
- Hypersensitivity to cyclosporine
- Live vaccinations
- Active infections and poorly controlled diabetes
- Concomitant drugs affecting cyclosporine pharmacokinetics
- Concurrent methotrexate administration
- Pregnancy and lactation
- Alcohol and drug abuse.

Toxicity

Presence of any of the following features is indicative of the toxicity/overdosage of cyclosporine:

Renal impairment, increasing glomerular fibrosis with increasing duration of treatment with higher dosages, hypertension, malignancies especially cutaneous squamous cell carcinoma, headache, tremor, paresthesias, hypertrichosis, gingival hyperplasia, worsening of acne, nausea/vomiting/diarrhea, myalgias, flu-like symptoms, lethargy, hypertriglyceridemia, hypomagnesemia, hyperkalemia, hyperbilirubinemia and increased risk of Infections.

Drug Interactions

- Concurrent methotrexate administration
- Inducers/Inhibitors of cytochrome P450 3A4
- St John's Wort decreases cyclosporine concentration
- Cyclosporine may reduce clearance of digoxin, colchicine, prednisolone, statins (increased risk of rhabdomyolysis)
- Potassium-sparing diuretics cause hyperkalemia
- Thiazide diuretics increase nephrotoxicity
- Killed vaccines may have decreased efficacy
- Live vaccination is contraindicated.

Precyclosporine screening/baseline monitoring should include:

It is recommended that a thorough history and physical examination (including blood pressure measurement) should be done at baseline to exclude contraindications.

- Measurement of blood pressure, CBC, LFT, KFT, urinalysis, lipid profile, serum magnesium, uric acid, and pregnancy test if indicated are recommended at baseline.

Ongoing Monitoring

It is recommended that blood pressure, BUN and serum creatinine should be repeated every other week during the initial 3 months, and thereafter at 1-monthly intervals.

- CBC, LFT, lipid profile, magnesium, uric acid, and potassium should be done at monthly intervals
- Pregnancy testing if indicated.

Note

- Estimating creatinine clearance (mL/minute): Cockcroft and Gault equation:
- CrCl = (140-age) × IBW/(Scr × 72)(× 0.85 for females).
- IBW–Ideal body weigaht.
- IBW in males = 50 kg+2.3 kg for each inch over 5 feet.
- IBW in females = 45.5 kg+2.3 kg for each inch over 5 feet.
- CSA—Cyclosporin.
- BUN—Blood urea nitrogen; CBC—Complete blood count; LFT—Liver function test.t

Points to Remember

- Cyclosporine (CSA) has the highest efficacy among all the nonbiologic systemic therapies. It is called the crisis drug as it is effective in cases resistant to other modalities and brings rapid control even in very severe cases
- Cyclosprine cannot be used at the same time with psoralen + UVA (PUVA) or UVB phototherapy, methotrexate or other immunosuppressive agents, coal tar, or radiation therapy
- CSA should be given in intermittent courses of maximum 12 weeks duration due to risk of renal damage. Another concern with CSA is the increased incidence of cutaneous squamous cell carcinomas

REFERENCES

1. Mueller W, Herrman B. Cyclosporin A for psoriasis (Letter). N Engl J Med 1979;301:555.
2. Marks JM. Cyclosporin A treatment of severe psoriasis (Letter). Br J Dermatol 1986;115:745-6.
3. Jegasothy BV, Ackerman CD, Todo S. Tacrolimus(FK506): a new therapeutic agent for severe recalcitrant psoriasis. Arch Dermatol. 1992;128:781-5.
4. Gottlieb AB, Griffiths CEM, Ho VC, et al. Oral pimecrolimus in the treatment of moderate to severe plaque type psoriasis: a double-blind multicentre, randomized, dose finding study. Br J Dermatol 2005;152:1219-27.
5. Marsland AM, Griffiths CEM. The macrolide immuno-suppressants in dermatology: mechanisms of action. Eur J Dermatol. 2002;12:618-22.
6. Kapoor R, Kapoor JR. Cyclosporine resolves generalized pustular psoriasis Arch Dermatol. 2006;142:1373-75.
7. Reynolds NJ, Al-Daraji WI. Calcineurin inhibitors and sirolimus: mechanism of action and applications in dermatology. Clin Exp Dermatol. 2002;27:555-61.
8. Berth-Jones J, Voorhees JJ. Consensus conference on cyclosporine A microemulsion for psoriasis. Br J Dermatol. 1996;135:775-7.
9. Wentzell JM, Baughman RD, O'Conner GT, et al. Cyclosporin in the treatment of psoriasis(Letter). Arch Dermatol. 1987;123:163-5.
10. Paul C, HO VC, McGeown C, et al. Risk of malignancies in psoriasis patients treated with cyclosporine: a 5 year cohort study. J Invest Dermatol 2003;120:211-6.
11. Heyendael VM, Spuls PI, Tenberge IJ, et al. Cyclosporine trough levels: is monitoring necessary during short-term treatment in psoriasis? A systematic review and clinical data on trough levels. Br J Dermatol. 2002;147:122-9.

Chapter

21 Methotrexate in Psoriasis

Strength of recommendation—B
Level of evidence—II
Pregnancy category status-Category—X.

Methotrexate is a stable analogue of aminopterin which may be given orally, intramuscularly, subcutaneously or intravenously. Methotrexate (MTX) is a gold standard systemic drug in the treatment of psoriasis. Despite the insurgence of various biologic therapies, MTX still is the mainstay of treatment either as monotherapy or in combination with other drugs. Until recently, it was widely believed that the folate metabolism antagonism is the main mechanism of action of methotrexate in psoriasis. However, the results of recent in vitro studies suggest that MTX causes inhibition of 5-aminoimidazole-4-carboxamide ribonucleotide (AICAR) transformylase leading to accumulation of AICAR, which in turn causes increased tissue concentration of adenosine (an antiinflammatory agent). The anti-inflammatory properties of adenosine are believed to decrease T-cell mediated inflammation in psoriasis and hence the improvement in disease control.[1]

DOSING AND ADMINISTRATION

Methotrexate is administered as a weekly single oral dose. Intramuscular administration is helpful when there is gastrointestinal intolerance to oral dosing or if there are concerns regarding patient compliance. Subcutaneous injection is equally effective and can be self-administered at home. Although there are no established maximum or minimum dosages of MTX, weekly dosages usually range from 7.5–25 mg given orally or parenterally. Most of the studies reported in literature have used MTX starting at lower doses (7.5 mg/week) and gradually escalating the dose according to the response. Doses can be increased gradually until an optimal response is achieved. The total dose should not ordinarily exceed 30 mg/week and the dose should be reduced to the lowest possible amount of drug needed to achieve adequate control of psoriasis with concomitant topical therapy.

American academy of dermatology recommends a test dose of 2.5–5 mg in those who are at risk of hematologic toxicity and with decreased calculated glomerular filtration rate.

Duration of Dosing

Treatment can be continued for as long as necessary provided there are no meaningful signs of liver or bone-marrow toxicity with adequate monitoring. Folic acid supplementation

1–5 mg daily by mouth, except for the day of methotrexate dosing, reduces the frequency of side-effects.[2,3]

Advantages and Benefits of Methotrexate

Following are some of the main benefits of methotrexate use:

- It is reasonably effective, is characterized by convenient dosing and is relatively inexpensive
- Improvements are noticeable following 6–8 weeks of therapy
- Methotrexate can be used for longer periods of time in comparison with other agents (such as cyclosporine), but patients must be regularly monitored for potentially serious side-effects
- Methotrexate can also enhance the effect of UVB phototherapy.

Risks and Side-effects

The adverse effects associated with the use of methotrexate include nausea, vomiting, epigastric discomfort, headache, skin irritation, hair loss, mouth ulcers, fatigue and low white blood cell count. The long-term risks include birth defects, kidney damage, bone marrow toxicity, and bone marrow suppression (rare, but potentially life-threatening). Long-term MTX use can cause serious liver damage. Routine blood tests assessing hepatic function may not detect the damage, hence, a liver biopsy may be necessary every 1.5–2 years while undergoing treatment.

Methotrexate can cause birth defects and miscarriages, hence women with childbearing potential taking the drug must use a reliable method of contraception.

To mitigate the risk of liver damage, patients must be advised not to consume alcohol while on therapy.[4,5]

Recommendations for Methotrexate

Indications

- Severe, recalcitrant, disabling psoriasis that is not adequately responsive to other forms of therapy
- Eythrodermic psoriasis
- Pustular psoriasis (generalized or localized)
- Psoriatic arthritis
- Severe nail psoriasis
- Psoriasis not responding to topical treatment, photochemotherapy and/or systemic retinoids.

Contraindications to the use of Methotrexate

Absolute Contraindications

The absolute contraindications to the use of methotrexate include:

- Hypersensitivity to methotrexate, pregnancy, lactation, severe and active infections, peptic ulcer (active), significantly reduced pulmonary function, concomitant intake of drugs that

increase MTX levels such as cotrimoxazole, alcoholic liver disease, hepatitis, severe fibrosis, cirrhosis and excessive alcohol intake, immunodeficiency syndromes, bone-marrow hypoplasia, leukopenia, thrombocytopenia or significant anemia
- Men and women considering conception should be off methotrexate for 3 months before attempting to conceive; and should pregnancy ensue before this time period, consider genetic counseling
- Mothers receiving methotrexate should not breastfeed.

Relative Contraindications

The relative contraindications to the use of methotrexate include: Abnormalities in renal function (creatinine clearance <60 mL/minute), abnormalities in liver function, obesity and diabetes mellitus.

Features Suggestive of Methotrexate Toxicity

- Presence of the following features are suggestive of methotrexate toxicity: Nausea, vomiting, diarrhea, malaise or fatigue, chills and fever, ulcerative stomatitis, dizziness, decreased resistance to infection, gastrointestinal (GI) ulceration and bleeding, photosensitivity ("radiation recall") and alopecia
- Elevated liver function test (LFT) results. Minor elevations of LFT results are common; if elevation exceeds twice normal, LFT must be checked more frequently. If it exceeds three times normal, consider dose reduction and if it exceeds 5 times normal, discontinue methotrexate
- Anemia, aplastic anemia, leukopenia and thrombocytopenia
- Interstitial pneumonitis.

Evidence of efficacy: In the only placebo-controlled trial of methotrexate for psoriasis, 36% of patients treated with 7.5 mg/week orally, increased as needed up to 25 mg/week, reached Psoriasis Area and Severity Index (PASI) 75 after 16 week. In recent comparative efficacy studies, MTX was found to have slightly lower efficacy compared to cyclosporine A (CSA). The drug has also been reported to be safe and effective in childhood psoriasis. Recently, the efficacy of MTX has been compared with biologics in the treatment of psoriasis. In a double-blind placebo-controlled study of MTX versus adalimumab, 250 patients were randomized into three subgroups receiving MTX or adalimumab or placebo. MTX was given in doses of 7.5 mg weekly, increased as needed to 25 mg per week. At week 16, PASI 75 was achieved by 19% in the placebo arm, 36% in the MTX group and 80% in the adalimumab group. In addition, MTX has been used as a combination therapy with many biologic agents approved by FDA. The combination therapy increases the efficacy and decreases the dose of individual drug, thereby decreasing the side-effects. Specific advantage of combining tumor necrosis factor inhibitors (infliximab) with MTX has been the suppression of neutralizing autoantibodies formation. The drug has been combined with etanercept, when the efficacy of etanercept monotherapy is insufficient. Alefacept has been used with MTX for psoriatic arthritis patients mostly with good results.[5]

Methotrexate is approved for the treatment of juvenile rheumatoid arthritis. Low-dose methotrexate has been used effectively and safely in children for a variety of dermatologic and rheumatologic disorders.

Although there are only two small controlled trials evaluating methotrexate for psoriatic arthritis that are inadequately powered to assess clinical benefit, methotrexate is often used as the primary agent to treat psoriatic arthritis.[6,7,8]

Folic acid supplementation and methotrexate use: The use of folic acid supplementation in patients on methotrexate has been a controversial issue, as various studies have reported that folic acid decreases the efficacy of methotrexate. Its use is advocated to limit the toxicity of MTX on liver, blood cells and gastrointestinal tract but there is a concern that it might reduce the efficacy of MTX. One of the main advantages of folic acid supplementation is believed to be a decrease in the incidence of gastrointestinal side effects. Prey et al. conducted a systematic review to find out the effect of folic and folinic acid supplementation on MTX associated toxicity and efficacy in inflammatory diseases. They concluded that the folic acid supplementation is an effective measure to reduce the hepatic adverse effects. Gastrointestinal side effects were also lesser in those who received folic acid but the difference from the control group was not statistically significant.[4]

When to do a liver Biopsy?

- Patients at low risk—at baseline, biopsy is not necessary
- First biopsy: 3.5–4 g; subsequent biopsies to be considered after every 1.5 g cumulative dose
- Patients at high risk including history of diabetes, obesity, abnormal LFT results, excessive alcohol ingestion, chronic liver disease, family history of heritable liver disease. Consider baseline biopsy or at 6 months with subsequent biopsies after 1–1.5 g.

Pre-methotrexate screening/Baseline monitoring:[9,10] Before starting methotrexate in a patient it is recommended that a thorough history and physical examination should be done to exclude contraindications. Complete blood cell (CBC), platelet count, blood urea nitrogen (BUN), serum creatinine, LFT, mantoux test, chest radiograph (if patient has underlying pulmonary disease), pregnancy test and test for human immunodeficiency virus (HIV) in selected patients should be done at baseline.

Baseline liver biopsy is only indicated in patients with a history of significant liver disease.

Ongoing Monitoring

It is recommended that CBC and platelet counts should be repeated initially every 2–4 weekly for first few months and then every 1–3 monthly depending on dosage adjustments, symptoms, and previous CBC count results.

- LFT should be repeated at monthly intervals, while KFT should be repeated every 2–3 monthly depending on dosage adjustments, symptoms and previous results
- Pregnancy test if indicated
- Consider liver biopsy in patients at high risk including history of diabetes, obesity, abnormal LFT results, excessive alcohol ingestion, chronic liver disease and family history of heritable liver disease. For those without risk factors, consider liver biopsy when cumulative dose reaches more than 3.5–4 g methotrexate
- For patients without risk factors, consider repeated liver biopsies after each subsequent 1.5 g dosage, based on LFT results, risk factors (e.g. diabetes and obesity) or in consultation with a hepatologist

- The aminoterminal peptide of procollagen III is used in Europe (but is generally not available in the United States) as a test for hepatic fibrosis, reducing the need for frequent liver biopsies.

Monitoring for Hepatotoxicity in Patients with No Risk Factors for Hepatotoxicity

- No baseline liver biopsy is needed
- Monitor liver function test (LFT) results monthly for the first 6 months and then every 1-3 months thereafter
- For elevations <2-fold upper limit of normal: repeat in 2–4 weeks
- For elevations >2-fold but <3-fold upper limit of normal: closely monitor, repeat in 2–4 weeks, and decrease dose as needed
- For persistent elevations in aspartate aminotransferase (AST) and alanine aminotransferase (ALT) levels during a 12-month period or if there is a decline in the serum albumin below the normal range with normal nutritional status, in a patient with well-controlled disease, a liver biopsy should be performed
- Consider liver biopsy after 3.5–4.0 g total cumulative dosage

Or

- Consider switching to another agent or discontinuing therapy after 3.5–4.0 g total cumulative dosage

Or

- Consider continuing to follow-up according to above guidelines without biopsy.

Monitoring for Hepatotoxicity in Patients with Risk Factors for Hepatotoxicity

- Consider the use of a different systemic agent
- Consider delayed baseline liver biopsy (after 2–6 months of therapy to establish medication efficacy and tolerability)
- Repeated liver biopsies after approximately 1–1.5 g of methotrexate are recommended.

Grading and Staging of Liver Biopsy

The liver biopsy is the best test we have today for finding out if the liver is healthy or damaged.

There are a variety of ways to interpret a liver biopsy. The most common scoring methods include Metavir and histologic activity index (HAI) also called the Knodell. It is important to remember that the length of the liver specimen and the knowledge of the professional reading the biopsy can influence the interpretation of the report.

Metavir Scoring System[11]

The Metavir scoring system was especially designed for patients with hepatitis C. The scoring consists of using a grading and a staging system. The grade gives an indication of the activity or amount of inflammation and the stage represents the amount of fibrosis or scarring. The grade is assigned a number based on the degree of inflammation, which is usually scored from 0-4 with 0 being no activity and 3 or 4 considered severe activity. The amount of inflammation is important because it is considered a precursor to fibrosis.

The fibrosis score is also assigned a number from 0-4.
0 = No scarring
1 = Minimal scarring
2 = Scarring has occurred and extends outside the areas in the liver that contains blood vessels
3 = Bridging fibrosis is spreading and connecting to other areas that contain fibrosis
4 = Cirrhosis or advanced scarring of the liver.

Knodell Scoring System[12]

The Knodell score or histologic activity index (HAI) is also commonly used to stage liver disease. It is a somewhat more complex process, but some experts believe that it is a better tool for defining the extent of liver inflammation and damage. It is composed of four individually assigned numbers that make up a single score. The first component (perioportal and/or bridging necrosis) is scored 0–10. The next two components (intralobular degeneration and portal inflammation) are scored 0–4. The combination of these three markers indicates the amount of inflammation in the liver:
0 = no inflammation
1–4 = minimal inflammation
5–8 = mild inflammation
9–12 = moderate inflammation
13–18 = marked inflammation

The fourth component indicates the amount of scarring in the liver and is scored from 0 (no scarring) to 4 (extensive scarring or cirrhosis). Information about the grade and stage of liver disease is helpful for the healthcare provider and the patient in guiding medical management. For example, treatment is usually indicated if the Metavir score is greater than or equal to 2 or the Ishak/Knodell score is greater than or equal to 3. For people with moderate to severe liver damage it is generally recommended that a more aggressive treatment approach is warranted. For people with a milder form of liver disease a watch and wait approach is usually recommended.

Note: MTX-Methotrexate; CBC—Complete blood count; LFT—Liver function test.

Points to Remember

- Methotrexate is a gold standard drug in the management of psoriasis even in the era of biologicals
- The utility of folic acid (FA) supplementation with MTX use is debatable. Its use is advocated to limit the toxicity of MTX on liver, blood cells and gastrointestinal tract but there is a concern that it might reduce the efficacy of MTX
- MTX causes inhibition of 5-aminoimidazole-4-carboxamide ribonucleotide (AICAR) transformylase leading to accumulation of AICAR, which in turn causes increased tissue concentration of adenosine. Primarily, this increased tissue concentration of adenosine accounts for its anti-inflammatory properties leading to symptom alleviation in psoriasis

REFERENCES

1. Kalb RE, Strober B, Weinstein G, Lebwohl M. Methotrexate and psoriasis: 2009 National Psoriasis Foundation consensus conference. J Am Acad Dermatol. 2009;60:824-37.
2. Weinstein GD. Commentary: three decades of folic acid antagonist in dermatology. Arch Dermatol. 1983;119:525-7.
3. Van Scott EJ, Auerbach R, Weinstein G. Parenteral methotrexate in psoriasis. Arch Dermatol. 1964;89:550-6.
4. Kirby B, Lyon CC, Griffiths CEM, Chalmers RJG. The use of folic acid supplementation in psoriasis patients receiving methotrexate: a survey in the United Kingdom. Clin Dermatol. 2000;25:265-8.
5. Saurat JH, Stingl G, Dubertret L, et al. Efficacy and safety results from the randomised controlled comparative study of adalimumab vs methotrexate vs placebo in patients with psoriasis. Br J Dermatol. 2008;158:558-66.
6. Roenigk HH Jr, Fowler B W, Curtis GH. Methotrexate for psoriasis in weekly oral doses. Arch Dermatol. 1969;99:86-93.
7. Kaur S, Kaur I, Bhushnurmath SR, et al. Methotrexate therapy for psoriasis (A preliminary report). Ind J Dermatol Venereol. 1986;52:155-7.
8. Nyfors A. Methotrexate therapy for psoriasis effect and side effects with particular reference to hepatic changes: A Survey. Aarhus, Denmark, Laegeforeningens Forlag. 1980.
9. Barker J, Horn EJ, Lebwohl M, Warren RB, Nast A, Rosenberg W, et al. Assessment and management of methotrexate hepatotoxicity in psoriasis patients: Report from a consensus conference to evaluate current practice and identify key questions toward optimizing methotrexate use in the clinic. J Eur Acad Dermatol Venereol. 2011;25:758-64.
10. Van Dooren-Greebe RJ, Kujipers ALA, Mulder J. Methotrexate revisited: effects of long term treatment in psoriasis. Br J Dermatol. 1994;130:204-10.
11. Newman M, Auerbach R, Feiner H, Holzman RS, Shupack J, Migdal P, et al. The role of liver biopsies in psoriatic patients receiving long-term methotrexate treatment. Improvement in liver abnormalities after cessation of treatment. Arch Dermatol. 1989;125:1218-24.
12. Maurice PD, Maddox AJ, Green CA, Tatnall F, Schofield JK, Stott DJ. Monitoring patients on methotrexate: Hepatic fibrosis not seen in patients with normal serum assays of aminoterminal peptide of type III procollagen. Br J Dermatol. 2005;152:451-8.

Chapter

22

Azathioprine in Psoriasis

Strength of recommendation—C
Level of evidence—III
Pregnancy category status—D

Azathioprine is a synthetic purine analogue which is synthesized by attaching 6-mercaptopurine to an imidazole ring. In-vivo it is converted to its active metabolite 6-mercaptopurine by hepatic xanthine oxidase. Azathioprine is an immunosuppressant used in the treatment of blistering disorders, atopic dermatitis and various inflammatory dermatoses. There are no randomized controlled clinical trials but few open label studies suggest its efficacy in psoriasis. There are some recent reports to suggest that this drug could be a good choice in psoriasis patients with concurrent bullous pemphigoid. Azathioprine acts slowly requiring at least 6–8 weeks for the onset of action. Important adverse effects include myelosuppression, liver toxicity and gastrointestinal side effects. Thiopurine methyltransferase (TPMT) levels should be measured to guide dosing. There is no FDA-approved use of azathioprine for psoriasis.[1,2] One suggested daily schedule guided by results of TPMT values is (table below):

TPMT <5.0 U—Do not use azathioprine
TPMT 5–13.7 U—Up to 0.5 mg/kg max dose
TPMT 13.7–19.0 U—Up to 1.5 mg/kg max dose
TPMT >19.0 U—Up to 2.5 mg/kg max dose.

Alternatively, start at 0.5 mg/kg and monitor for cytopenia. If no cytopenia occurs, increase the dose by 0.5 mg/kg/day after 6–8 weeks if necessary and increase by 0.5 mg/kg/day every 4 weeks thereafter as needed. It is generally dosed at 75–150 mg/day.

Evidence of efficacy and safety: In one study 19/29 patients had >75% improvement but in another smaller study 5/10 patients had >25% improvement. A small observational cohort study suggests that azathioprine may be of value in psoriatic arthritis.

CONTRAINDICATIONS

Absolute

- Hypersensitivity to azathioprine
- Pregnancy or attempting pregnancy
- Active and severe infections

- Pregnancy and breastfeeding should be avoided during treatment with azathioprine, and patients (including males) must use adequate contraception.

Relative

- Concurrent use of allopurinol
- Prior treatment with cyclophosphamide or chlorambucil.

Adverse Effects

Features suggesting toxicity or overdosage are as follows: Vomiting, diarrhea, frequent infections, pancreatitis, hepatitis, bone-marrow suppression and development of malignancies (cutaneous squamous cell carcinoma, lymphoproliferative malignancies).

DRUG INTERACTIONS

- Concurrent use of azathioprine with allopurinol, captopril and cotrimoxazole increases risk of hematologic toxicity
- Concurrent use of azathioprine with warfarin and pancuronium may need an increased dose of warfarin and pancuronium for their optimal action
- Rifampicin—decreases azathioprine efficacy, besides being also hepatotoxic
- Clozapine—increased risk of agranulocytosis.

Preazathioprine screening/Baseline monitoring should include:
It is recommended that a thorough history and physical examination should be done at baseline to exclude contraindications to the use of azathioprine. CBC, DLC, LFT, KFT, urinalysis, Mantoux test, hepatitis B and C screen and pregnancy test (if indicated) should be done at baseline.

CBC count/differential count should then be repeated twice monthly for the first 2 months, and repeated monthly for the next 2 months followed by every 2 months thereafter.

LFT should be done monthly for the first 3 months and then repeated every 2 months thereafter.

A six monthly general physical examination focusing on lymph node examination and skin cancer examination (SCCs in particular) is also recommended while the patient is on azathioprine.[3,4,5]

Note: TPMT—Thiopurine methyl transferase; CBC—Complete blood count; DLC—Differential leucocyte count; LFT—Liver function test.

Points to Remember

- ❖ Azathioprine is an immunosuppressant used in the treatment of blistering disorders, atopic dermatitis and various inflammatory dermatoses
- ❖ There are no randomized trials but few open label studies suggest its efficacy in psoriasis
- ❖ There is no FDA-approved use of azathioprine for psoriasis
- ❖ Ideally, TPMT levels should be done prior to the use of azathioprine

REFERENCES

1. Du Vivier A, Munro DD, Verbov J. Treatment of psoriasis with azathioprine. Br Med J 1974;1:49-51.
2. Greaves MW, Dawber R. Azathioprine in psoriasis. Br Med J 1970;2:237-8.
3. Roeder C, Driesch PV. Psoriatic erythroderma and bullous pemphigoid treated successfully with acitretin and azathioprine. Eur J Dermatol 1999;9:537-9.
4. Snow JL, Gibson LE. The role of genetic variation in thiopurine methyltransferase activity and the efficacy and/or side effects of azathioprine therapy in dermatologic patients. Arch Dermatol 1995;131:193-7.
5. Hacker SM, Ramos-Caro FA, Ford MJ, Flowers FP. Azathiopurine: a forgotten alternative for treatment of severe psoriasis.Int J Dermatol 1992;31:873-4.

Chapter

23 Fumaric Acid Esters

Strength of recommendation—B
Level of evidence—I
Pregnancy category status—No FDA pregnancy category status.

Fumaric acid esters (FAE) are a mixture of dimethylfumarate (DMF) and calcium, magnesium and zinc salts of monoethylfumaric acid commonly used in Northern Europe, particularly in Germany and Netherlands, as the first line systemic treatment for moderate to severe psoriasis, with proven efficacy and low toxicity. The mechanism of action of the drug is only partially understood. Lehmann et al. in an in vitro assay found that DMF and diethylfumarate are the active compounds and FAEs mediates its immunomodulatory activity by the induction of the anti-inflammatory stress protein, heme oxygenase 1. It is given in doses of 120–720 mg (DMF) daily. The starting dose is one tablet of Fumaderm which is then increased over the next 8 weeks to a maximum of 6 tablets daily. There is no FDA approved use of FAEs for psoriasis in the United States, but are approved in Europe for the treatment of psoriasis.

Recent studies suggest that FAEs are effective as monotherapy and can be used in combination with other oral antipsoriatic agents. Subjective side-effects are mainly gastrointestinal and flushing. The drug does not affect the liver and renal functions significantly but lymphopenia is a common adverse effect which needs close monitoring.[1,2]

EVIDENCE OF EFFICACY AND SAFETY

A multicenter, randomized, double-blind placebo-controlled trial of 100 patients showed that after 16 weeks, patients treated with fumarates reached a mean PASI 50 compared with patients given placebo whose PASI was essentially unchanged. Balasubramaniam et al. from United Kingdom reported good efficacy and safety of FAEs, both as monotherapy and in combination therapy with cyclosporine, acitretin, hydroxyurea and methotrexate. In an another nonrandomized prospective cohort study, 80 patients with severe, recalcitrant, chronic plaque psoriasis received FAEs. Of the total patients, 59% were on other concomitant oral antipsoriatic agent. At 3 months, PASI 90 was achieved in 4%, PASI 75 in 8% and PASI 50 in 20% of cases. Side effects were reported by 74% of patients, resulting in cessation of FAEs in 36% of cases. Most common side effects were diarrhea, abdominal pain and flushing, whereas lymphopenia occurred in 33% of patients.

Reich et al. analyzed the data of 984 patients who were treated with FAEs for at least 24 months (mean duration 44 months). There was marked improvement in 67% after 6 months, 78% after 24 months, and 82% of patients after 36 months of therapy. Changes of laboratory parameters were usually insignificant. Case series of patients treated up to 14 years suggest no increased risk for infections or malignancies, however large, long-term follow-up studies are necessary to confirm these observations.[3,4]

CONTRAINDICATIONS

The contraindications to the use of fumaric acid esters include: Severe liver disease, severe or chronic GI disease, severe or chronic kidney disease, malignancy or a history of malignancy, leukopenia and other hematologic abnormalities, pregnancy and breastfeeding. Other fumaric acid derivatives, methotrexate, cyclosporine, immunosuppressive drugs, and cytostatic drugs may potentiate toxicity,when given along with fumarates.

Drugs known to cause renal dysfunction should not be used concurrently with fumarates.

SIDE EFFECTS

The adverse effects which have been reported with the use of FAEs are gastrointestinal (abdominal cramps, nausea, diarrhea, fullness, and flatulence), flushing, malaise, fatigue, lymphopenia, leukopenia, eosinophilia, hepatotoxicity and elevated LFT results, increased cholesterol, triglycerides, increased serum creatinine and potassium, and proteinuria. There are rare case reports of renal disease but none have been reported in the controlled trials.

MONITORING OF PATIENTS ON FUMARATES

At baseline before putting patients on FAEs, it is recommended that a thorough history and physical examination should be done along with investigations which include CBC, platelet count, LFT, KFT and urine analysis. It is recommended that CBC and platelet counts should be repeated every other week for the first 2 months, followed monthly until 6 months and bimonthly thereafter.

Serum chemistry and urinalysis should be repeated every 2 weeks for the first month, then monthly for the first 6 months and bimonthly thereafter.[5]

Note: FAE—Fumaric acid esters; CBC—Complete blood count; LFT—Liver function test.

Points to Remember

- There is no FDA approved use of fumarates in psoriasis
- These are used in Northern Europe, particularly in Germany and Netherlands, as the first line systemic treatment for moderate to severe psoriasis, with proven efficacy and low toxicity

REFERENCES

1. Wain EM, Darling MI, Pleass RD, Barker JN, Smith CH. Treatment of severe, recalcitrant, chronic plaque psoriasis with fumaric acid esters: A prospective study. Br J Dermatol. 2010;162:427-34.
2. Balasubramaniam P, Stevenson O, Berth-Jones J. Fumaric acid esters in severe psoriasis, including experience of use in combination with other systemic modalities. Br J Dermatol. 2004;150:741-6.
3. Reich K, Thaci D, Mrowietz U, Kamps A, Neureither M, Luger T. Efficacy and safety of fumaric acid esters in the long-term treatment of psoriasis—a retrospective study (FUTURE) J Dtsch Dermatol Ges. 2009;7:603-11.
4. Yazdi MR, Mrowietz U. Fumaric acid esters. Clin Dermatol. 2008;26:522-56.
5. Mrowietz U, Christophers E, Altemeyer P. Treatment of psoriasis with fumaric acid esters: results of a prospective multicentre study. German Multicentre study. Br J Dermatol. 1998;138:456-60.

Chapter

24 Hydroxyurea in Psoriasis

Strength of recommendation—C
Level of evidence—III
Pregnancy category status—D

Hydroxycarbamide (hydroxyurea) is an antimetabolite that has been used principally for the treatment of malignant diseases, particularly chronic myeloid leukemia. Hydroxyurea is an antimetabolite which works by inhibiting DNA replication. Its efficacy in psoriasis is known for 30 years. However, the drug has not been extensively used in psoriasis. The active drug which is converted invivo from its parent, blocks the conversion of ribonucleotides to deoxyribonucleotides by interfering with the enzyme ribonucleoside diphosphate reductase, thereby inhibiting DNA synthesis in proliferating cells. There is a renewed interest in its use from India. There is no FDA-approved use for psoriasis. It is given in an initial dose of 500 mg orally twice daily, increasing to up to 3 g/day as tolerated. A dose of 3–4.5 g/week has also been used. It provides a useful cheap alternative for systemic treatment of psoriasis.

EVIDENCE OF EFFICACY

The drug has not been extensively used in psoriasis. The efficacy rates vary widely. Kumar et al. treated 31 patients of chronic plaque psoriatics with 1–1.5 g daily doses of hydroxyurea. Greater than 50% patients showed more than 70% reduction in PASI score. Sharma et al. used hydroxyurea in 34 psoriatic patients with similar results. In a recent comparative study of methotrexate and hydroxyurea, there was 77% and 49% reduction in the mean PASI score, respectively, at 12 weeks. Gach et al. used hydroxyurea in combination with infliximab to treat a recalcitrant case of psoriasis. One study found that 60% of 85 patients treated for a mean of 16 months had a complete or almost complete clearance.

SIDE EFFECTS

The adverse effects which have been reported with the use of hydroxyurea inclue fever, chills, malaise, edema, asthenia, elevation of hepatic enzymes, bone-marrow suppression, GI symptoms (stomatitis, anorexia, nausea, vomiting, diarrhea and constipation), dermatologic reactions (rash, ulceration, dermatomyositis-like skin changes, alopecia), dysuria, neurologic disturbances (headache, dizziness, disorientation, hallucinations and convulsions), temporary impairment of renal tubular function accompanied by elevations in serum uric acid, BUN and creatinine and pulmonary fibrosis rarely. Fatal and nonfatal pancreatitis and hepatotoxicity and severe peripheral neuropathy have been reported in HIV-infected patients who received hydroxyurea in combination with antiretroviral agents.[1-3]

CONTRAINDICATIONS

Marked bone-marrow depression, including leukopenia, thrombocytopenia and/or anemia are absolute contraindications to the use of hydroxyurea. Concurrent use of hydroxyurea and other myelosuppressive agents or radiation therapy may increase the likelihood of bone-marrow depression. Hydroxyurea may raise the serum uric acid level; dosage adjustment of uricosuric medication may thus be necessary. Pregnancy and breastfeeding should be avoided during treatment and patients (including males) must use adequate contraception.

MONITORING

History and physical examination with focuss on lymphadenopathy and cutaneous cancer examination (SCCs in particular), CBC and pregnancy test if indicated should be done at baseline. CBC should then be repeated at monthly intervals. A six monthly physical examination focusing on lymph-node examination and skin-cancer examination (SCCs in particular) is recommended.[4-6]

Points to Remember

- There is no FDA approved use of hydroxyurea in psoriasis
- Hydroxyurea is primarily used in the treatment of CML
- Hydroxyurea is a promising systemic treatment option for psoriasis because of less adverse effects

Note: CBC—Complete blood count; BUN—Blood urea nitrogen; PASI—Psoriasis area severity index.

REFERENCES

1. Layton AM, Sheehan-Dare RA, Goodfield MJ, Cotterill JA. Hydroxyurea in the management of therapy resistant psoriasis. Br J Dermatol. 1989;121:647-53.
2. Kumar B, Saraswat A, Kaur I. Rediscovering hydroxyurea: its role in recalcitrant psoriasis. Int J Dermatol. 2001;40:530-4.
3. Sharma VK, Dutta B, Ramam M. Hydroxyurea as an alternative therapy for psoriasis. Indian J Dermatol Venereol Leprol. 2004;70:13-7.
4. Smith CH. Use of hydroxyurea in psoriasis. Clin Exp Dermatol. 1999;24:2-6.
5. Touraine R, Revuz J, Tulliez M. Psoriasis and hydroxyurea. Br J Dermatol. 1972;86:102.
6. Hunter GA, Simmons IJ, Thomas BM. A clinical trial of hydroxyurea for psoriasis. Australas J Dermatol. 1972;13:93-9.

Chapter

25 Leflunomide in Psoriasis

Strength of recommendation—B
Level of evidence—II
Pregnancy category status—X

Leflunomide, a pyrimidine synthesis inhibitor effective for rheumatoid arthritis, acts by inhibiting de novo pyrimidine synthesis. It is a disease-modifying antirheumatic drug which can be particularly beneficial for psoriasis patients with concurrent arthritis (PsA). There is no FDA-approved use of leflunomide for psoriasis.

EVIDENCE OF EFFICACY AND SAFETY

Leflunomide is given in a loading dose of 100 mg/day for 3 days followed by 20 mg/day. In the only randomized controlled trial of 190 patients, 24 weeks of leflunomide, dosed as above, led to a PASI 75 of 17% vs placebo response of 8% (P = .048). Psoriatic arthritis (PsA) responded in 59% in leflunomide group versus 30% in placebo group. Patients were allowed concurrent use of low-dose systemic corticosteroids for the treatment of their psoriatic arthritis. The long-term results are not reported with the use of leflunomide.

ADVERSE EFFECTS

The most common side effects include nausea, diarrhea, loss of appetite, weight loss, headache and dizziness. Less frequent adverse reactions may include severe liver injury, including fatal outcome (most cases of severe liver injury occur within 6 months of therapy and in patients with multiple risk factors for hepatotoxicity). Rare reports of pancytopenia, agranulocytosis, and thrombocytopenia in patients receiving leflunomide have been reported. But this occurs in patients who have been treated concurrently with methotrexate or other immunosuppressive agents, or who had recently discontinued these medications.[1,2]

CONTRAINDICATIONS

1. Patients with hypersensitivity to leflunomide or its metabolites.
2. Coadministration of leflunomide with methotrexate demonstrates no pharmacokinetic interaction between the two drugs but can lead to an increased risk of hepatotoxicity.
3. When leflunomide is given with rifampin, leflunomide levels are increased.
4. Leflunomide should not be used by nursing mothers.

MONITORING

A thorough history and physical examination with CBC, DLC, LFT and pregnancy test if indicated should be done at baseline. Subsequently it is recommended that CBC with differential count and LFT should be repeated monthly for the first 6 months and every 6–8 weeks thereafter.[3]

Points to Remember

Leflunomide, a pyrimidine synthesis inhibitor effective for rheumatoid arthritis, acts by inhibiting de novo pyrimidine synthesis. It is a disease-modifying antirheumatic drug which can be particularly beneficial for psoriasis patients with concurrent arthritis (PsA)

Note: PsA—Psoriatic arthritis; CBC—Complete blood count; DLC—Differential leucocyte count; LFT—Liver function test.

REFERENCES

1. Prakash A, Jarvis B. Leflunomide: A review of its use in active rheumatoid arthritis. Drugs. 1999;58:1137-64.
2. Kaltwasser JP, Nash P, Gladman D, Rosen CF, Behrens F, Jones P, et al. Efficacy and safety of leflunomide in the treatment of psoriatic arthritis and psoriasis: A multinational, double-blind, randomized, placebo-controlled clinical trial. Arthritis Rheum. 2004;50:1939-50.
3. Liang GC, Barr WG. Long term follow-up of the use of leflunomide in recalcitrant psoriatic arthritis and psoriasis.Arthritis Rheum. 2001;44(9S):S121.

Chapter

26

Mycophenolate Mofetil in Psoriasis

Strength of recommendation—C
Level of evidence—III
Pregnancy category status—D

Mycophenolate mofetil (MMF) is a prodrug of mycophenolic acid. It is a lymphocyte-selective immunosuppressive agent which acts by noncompetitive inhibition of de novo purine synthesis due to inhibition of inosine monophosphate dehydrogenase enzyme, thus resulting in blockade of T- and B-cell proliferation. MMF was first used for psoriasis in 1998. Subsequently, there are many reports suggesting the efficacy of MMF in psoriasis. This drug has been safely administered in HIV patients with psoriasis. MMF is a good choice in psoriasis patients concurrently suffering from immunobullous disorders. There is no FDA-approved use of MMF for psoriasis. It is usually given in a dose of 1–2 g daily in two divided doses.[1,2]

EVIDENCE OF EFFICACY AND SAFETY

Beissert et al. carried out a prospective, multicenter, randomized clinical trial comparing the efficacy of MMF with that of cyclosporine (CSA) for the treatment of chronic plaque-type psoriasis. After 12 weeks, CSA demonstrated a significantly superior efficacy compared to MMF but there was no difference in time to disease relapse, side effects and psoriasis disability index. In an another study of 23 patients who were treated with 1.0–1.5 g of MMF twice daily, a 47% mean reduction in PASI at 12 weeks was observed. In yet another study, a 47% mean reduction in PASI was observed at 6 weeks in 11 patients with psoriasis who were treated with 1 g MMF twice daily for 3 weeks, followed by 0.5 g twice daily for 3 more weeks.[1,2] The long-term results of MMF use in psoriasis are not known.

CONTRAINDICATIONS

Hypersensitivity to MMF and mycophenolic acid. Patients taking MMF should not be given live attenuated virus vaccines. Pregnancy and breastfeeding should be avoided during treatment and patients (including males) must use adequate contraceptive precautions. Antibiotics including cephalosporins, fluoroquinolones, macrolides, penems, penicillins, sulfonamides inhibit enterohepatic recirculation and decrease MMF levels, hence should not be given simultaneously.

SIDE EFFECTS

The side effects which are encountered with the use of MMF inclue fever and myalgias, headache, insomnia, peripheral edema, hypertension, GI side effects (diarrhea, nausea/vomiting, abdominal cramps), leukopenia, anemia and thrombocytopenia, genitourinary (urgency, frequency, dysuria, sterile pyuria), increased incidence of viral, bacterial and mycobacterial infections, progressive multifocal leukoencephalopathy, hypercholesterolemia, hypophosphatemia and hyper/hypokalemia.

Monitoring of Patients on Mycophenolate Mofetil

It is recommended that before putting patients on MMF, a thorough history and physical examination with focus on lymphadenopathy and any suspicious signs of cutaneous malignancy should be done. CBC, platelet count, KFT, LFT and pregnancy test if indicated should be done at baseline. It is recommended that CBC and platelet counts should be repeated weekly for 1 month; then every 2 weekly for 2 months; then monthly thereafter. LFT should be done at monthly intervals.

Six-monthly physical examination focusing on lymph-node examination and skin-cancer examination (SCCs in particular) is recommended.[3-5]

Points to Remember

- MMF is a lymphocyte-selective immunosuppressive agent which acts by noncompetitive inhibition of de novo purine synthesis due to inhibition of inosine monophosphate dehydrogenase enzyme, thus resulting in blockade of T- and B-cell proliferation
- There is no FDA-approved use of MMF for psoriasis

Note: MMF—Mycophenolate mofetil; CSA—Cyclosporine; CBC—Complete blood count; LFT—Liver function test; KFT—Kidney function test; PASI—Psoriasis area severity index.

REFERENCES

1. Haufs MG, Beissert S, Grabbe S, Schutte B, Luger TA. Psoriasis vulgaris treated successfully with mycophenolate mofetil. Br J Dermatol. 1998;138:179-81.
2. Zhou Y, Rosenthal D, Dutz F, Ho V. Mycophenolate mofetil (CellCept) for psoriasis: A two-center prospective open-label clinical trial. J Cutan Med Surg. 2003;7:193-7.
3. Geilen CC, Arnold M, Orfanos CE. Mycophenolate mofetil as a systemic antipsoriatic agent: Positive experience in 11 patients. Br J Dermatol. 2001;144:583-6.
4. Forman SB, Higginson R, Garrett AB. Psoriasis and psoriatic arthritis in a patient with HIV: Response to mycophenolate mofetil treatment. J Drugs Dermatol. 2008;7:972-3.
5. Grundmann-Kollmann M, Mooser G, Schraeder P. Treatment of chronic plaque-stage psoriasis and psoriatic arthritis with mycophenolate mofetil. J Am Acad Dermatol. 2000;45:835-7.

Chapter

27 Sulfasalazine in Psoriasis

Strength of recommendation—B
Level of evidence—II
Pregnancy category status—B

Sulfasalazine is an anti-inflammatory drug consisting of a combination of 5-aminosalicylic acid and sulfapyridine. Currently it is FDA approved for the treatment of ulcerative colitis and rheumatoid arthritis. There is no FDA-approved use for sulfasalazine in psoriasis. In psoriasis, it is started at an initial dose of 500 mg orally twice daily, which is then increased up to 3–4 g/day as tolerated. One of the benefits of sulfasalazine is that it can be given for prolonged periods as there are no known cumulative toxicities.

EVIDENCE OF EFFICACY AND SAFETY

The efficacy rates of sulfasalazine use in psoriasis are not well characterized; in an only randomized controlled clinical trial of sulfasalazine vs placebo, 8 weeks of 3–4 g/day sulfasalazine led to a moderate improvement in PASI in 7/17 patients (who received sulfasalazine) compared with 1/27 patients who recieved placebo. The long-term results have not been reported. In the largest trial of sulfasalazine for psoriatic arthritis, after 36 weeks of treatment with 2 g/day, 58% of patients given sulfasalazine compared with 45% of patients given placebo achieved control (Dougados et al., 1995).[1-3]

SIDE EFFECTS

Anorexia, headache, GI symptoms (including nausea, vomiting and gastric distress) and oligospermia can occur in up to one third of patients. Less frequent reactions include rash, pruritus, urticaria, fever, hemolytic anemia and cyanosis.

CONTRAINDICATIONS

Intestinal or urinary obstruction, patients with porphyria, hypersensitivity to sulfasalazine or its metabolites, sulfonamides and salicylates. Folic acid and digoxin should not be given simultaneously due to reduced absorption of these agents. Sulfonamides are excreted in the breast milk. In the newborn, they compete with bilirubin for binding sites on the plasma proteins and may thus, cause kernicterus. Thus, sulfasalazine should not be given to nursing mothers.

MONITORING

Baseline monitoring should consist of a thorough history and physical examination, CBC, LFT, KFT and pregnancy test if indicated. It is suggested that CBC and LFT should be repeated every other week for the first 3 months; and during the second 3 months, CBC and LFT monthly and thereafter once every 3 months. Renal function tests and urinanalysis should be done periodically.[4-6]

Sulfonamides are excreted in the breast milk. In the newborn, they compete with bilirubin for binding sites on the plasma proteins and may thus cause kernicterus.

Points to Remember

There is no FDA approved use of sulfasalazine in psoriasis. Currently it is FDA approved in the treatment of ulcerative colitis and rheumatoid arthritis

REFERENCES

1. Farr M. Sulphasalazine in psoriatic arthritis: double-blind placebo controlled study. Br J Rheumatol. 1993; 29: 46-9.
2. Fraser SM. Sulphasalazine in the management of psoriatic arthritis. Br J Rheumatol. 1993;32:923-25.
3. Stroehmann L. Therapy of seronegative oligoarthritis with salazopyrine. Z Rheumatol. 1987;46:79-82.
4. Gupta AK. Sulfasalazine: A potential psoriasis therapy? J Am Acad Dermatol. 1989;20:797-800.
5. Gupta AK. Sulfasalazine improves psoriasis: a double-blind analysia. J Am Acad Dermatol. 1990;126:487-93.
6. Watkinson G. Sulfasalazine: a review of 40 years' experience. Drugs. 1986;32:1-11.

Chapter

28 Tacrolimus in Psoriasis

Strength of recommendation—B
Level of evidence—II
Pregnancy category status—C

Tacrolimus is an immunosuppressive drug that is mainly used after allogenic-organ transplant to decrease the risk of graft rejection. It is used topically in dermatology for numerous indications. It is a macrolide lactone derived from the fermentation broth of a Japanese soil sample that contained the bacteria *Streptomyces tsukubaensis*. It reduces interleukin-2 (IL-2) production by T-cells.[1] There is no FDA-approved use of tacrolimus for psoriasis. It is given in a dose of 0.05–0.15 mg/kg, but the duration of dosing is unknown.

EVIDENCE OF EFFICACY

The efficacy rates of tacrolimus in psoriasis are poorly characterized;in one study patients who were given tacrolimus at a dose of 0.05 mg/kg showed no difference from placebo at 3 weeks;but when the dose was increased to 0.10–0.15 mg/kg, there was a statistically significant improvement in PASI compared with placebo at 9 weeks. However, the long-term results are not known.

SIDE EFFECTS

The most-common side effects of tacrolimus include tremor, headache, nausea, diarrhea, hypertension and abnormal renal function test results. The less-common side effects include hyperglycemia, hyperkalemia, elevated LFT results, anemia, leukocytosis, dyspnea, fever, arthralgias, edema, diabetes, insomnia and paresthesias.

CONTRAINDICATIONS

Patients with hypersensitivity to tacrolimus or its metabolites. Tacrolimus and cyclosporine should not be given together.

MONITORING OF PATIENTS ON TACROLIMUS

A proper history and physical examination including blood-pressure measurement should be done at baseline. CBC with TLC/DLC, KFT, LFT and pregnancy test if indicated are recommended at baseline. The proper frequency of ongoing monitoring has not been established.[2,3]

Points to Remember

- ❖ Tacrolimus is rarely used for the treatment of psoriasis, but is a useful alternative
- ❖ Tacrolimus is not FDA approved for psoriasis

Note: CBC—Complete blood count; DLC—Differential leucocyte count; LFT—Liver function test; KFT—Kidney function test.

REFERENCES

1. Jegasothy BV, Ackerman CD, Todo S, Fung JJ, Abu-Elmagd K, Starzl TE. Tacrolimus (FK 506) - a new therapeutic agent for severe recalcitrant psoriasis. Arch Dermatol. 1992;128:781-5.
2. Bos JD, Witkamp L, Zonnevald IM, Ruzicka T, Szarmach H, Szczerkowska-Dobosz A. Systemic tacrolimus (FK 506) is effective for the treatment of psoriasis in a double-blind, placebo-controlled study: The European FK 506 multicenter psoriasis study group. Arch Dermatol. 1996;132:419-23.
3. European FK506 Multicentre Psoriasis Study Group. Systemic tacrolimus (FK506) is effective for the treatment of psoriasis in a double-blind, placebo controlled study. Arch Dermatol. 1996;132:419-23.

Chapter

29 6-Thioguanine in Psoriasis

Strength of recommendation—C
Level of evidence—III
Pregnancy catergory status—D

6-Thioguanine belongs to the thiopurine family of drugs that also includes mercatopurine and azathiopurine, which are examples of antimetabolites. It is a purine analogue of the nucleobase guanine. It was primarily used for the treatment of ALL in children. There is no FDA-approved use for 6-thioguanine in psoriasis.[1,2] It is recommended to start it at dose of 80 mg twice a week, followed by an increase of 20 mg every 2–4 weeks to a maximum dose of 160 mg 3 times/week.

EVIDENCE OF EFFICACY

In an open-label trial of 14 patients who were treated with pulse dosing followed by maintenance dosage (120 mg twice/week to 160 mg 3 times/week);6 patients showed a response after 2–4 weeks, and 11 patients became longer-term responders. Another study showed that 14/18 patients had 90% improvement. It has been safely used up to 145 months.

There are no studies in psoriatic arthritis and pediatric psoriasis patients.

SIDE EFFECTS

The adverse effects which have been reported with the use of 6-thioguanine are headache, nausea, vomiting, taste disturbances, aphthous ulcers, fatigue, gastroesophageal reflux, gastric ulcers, myelosuppression, liver toxicity from hepatic veno-occlusive disease, increased alanine aminotransferase (ALT) and aspartate aminotransferase (AST) levels, hyperuricemia, photodermatitis and increased incidence of herpes zoster and warts.

CONTRAINDICATIONS TO THE USE OF 6-THIOGUANINE

Preexisting liver disease, immunosuppression, anemia, leukopenia and thrombocytopenia.

DRUG INTERACTIONS

Aminosalicylate derivatives (olsalazine, mesalazine and sulfasalazine) may inhibit thiopurine methyl transferase (TPMT) thus, increasing the serum levels of 6-thioguanine and potentiating toxicity.

HOW TO MONITOR PATIENTS ON 6-THIOGUANINE

It is recommended that at baseline, a thorough history and physical examination with focus on lymphadenopathy should be done. CBC, platelet count, serum creatinine, BUN, LFT, serology for hepatitis B and C, mantoux test and pregnancy test in females should be done. CBC and platelet counts should be repeated every 2–4 weeks and KFT every 3 monthly.

Note: It is recommended that biannual physical examination focusing on lymph-node examination and skin-cancer examination (SCCs in particular) should be performed while the patient is on 6-thioguanine.[3,4]

Points to Remember

- 6-Thiogaunine is not FDA approved for the treatment of psoriasis
- It is a useful alternative when other forms of treatment have failed

Note: CBC—Complete blood count; LFT—Liver function test; TPMT—Thiopurine methyl transferase.

REFERENCES

1. Zackheim HS, Maibach HI, Grekin DA. Thiogaunine for psoriasis. In: Farber EM, Cox AJ, Nail L, eds. Psoriasis. Proceedings of the third international symposium. New York: Grune & Stratton. 1982;405.
2. Ramagosa R, Kerdel F, Shah N. Treatment of psoriasis with 6-thiogaunine and hepatic veno-occlusive disease. J Am Acad Dermatol. 2002;47:970-2.
3. Molin L, Thomsen K. Thiogaunine treatment in psoriasis. Acta Derm Venereol. 1987;67:85-8.
4. Mason C, Kreuger GG. Thiogaunine for refractory psoriasis: a 4-year experience. J Am Acad Dermatol. 2001;44:67-72.

Chapter

30

Retinoic Acid Metabolism Blocking Agents in Psoriasis

Retinoic acid metabolism blocking agents (RAMBA) are retinoid mimetic drugs with a side effect profile similar to that of retinoids but of lower incidence. RAMBA act by blocking cytochrome P-450 dependent 4-hydroxylation of all-trans-retinoic acid (ATRA), thus modulating the intracellular levels of endogenous retinoids, leading to normalization of aberrant epithelial growth and differentiation, but the plasma ATRA levels do not rise beyond physiologic levels. These drugs have the advantage that they can be given more readily to women and children than retinoids as there is rapid clearance of the RAMBA unlike the available synthetic retinoids which may stay in the body for a long time. Liarazole and talarozole are RAMBAs which have been tried in psoriasis and found to be effective in some initial studies. Talarozole is a more selective inhibitor of the enzyme retinoic acid 4-hydroxylase, thus may allow the usage of reduced dose and hence fewer side effects. Talarozole is in phase II clinical trial stage.[1-3]

REFERENCES

1. Berth-Jones J, Todd G, Hutchinson PE, Thestrup-Pedersen K, Vanhoutte FP. Treatment of psoriasis with oral liarozole: a dose-ranging study. Br J Dermatol. 2000;143:1170-6.
2. Bhushan M, Burden AD, McElhone K, James R, Vanhoutte FP, Griffiths CE. Oral liarozole in the treatment of palmoplantar pustular psoriasis: A randomized, double-blind, placebo-controlled study. Br J Dermatol. 2001;145:546-53.
3. Geria AN, Scheinfeld NS. Talarozole, a selective inhibitor of P450-mediated all-trans retinoic acid for the treatment of psoriasis and acne. Curr Opin Investig Drugs. 2008;9:1228-37.

Chapter 31

Rapamycin Inhibitors: Sirolimus, Everolimus

Mammalian target of rapamycin (mTOR) is a protein kinase that controls cell growth, proliferation and survival. mTOR signaling is often upregulated in cancer and there is great interest in developing drugs that target this enzyme. Rapamycin and its analogs bind to a domain separate from the catalytic site to block a subset of mTOR functions. These drugs are extremely selective for mTOR and are already in clinical use for treating cancers, but they could potentially activate an mTOR-dependent survival pathway that could lead to treatment failure.

Sirolimus is similar in structure to cyclosporine (CSA) and tacrolimus, but it is not a calcineurin inhibitor. Sirolimus binds to FK506 binding protein12 (FKBP12) and interrupts the cell cycle progression from G1 to the S phase, leading to the suppression of T-lymphocyte activation and proliferation and hence, the possible beneficial effect in psoriasis. Sirolimus is believed to cause less nephrotoxicity, neurotoxicity and hypertension compared to CSA and tacrolimus. Sirolimus can be used in combination with CSA to limit the cumulative toxicity of both agents. Oral sirolimus, CSA and a combination of the two were assessed in a large multicenter study of 150 patients with severe chronic plaque psoriasis. Comparable results were obtained in patients treated with CSA alone (5.0 mg/kg/day) and in those treated with subtherapeutic CSA (1.25 mg/kg/day) combined with sirolimus (3.0 mg/m^2). Sirolimus monotherapy was found to be ineffective.[1]

Everolimus is a semisynthetic, immunosuppressive and antiproliferative macrolide derived from sirolimus and is believed to possess better pharmacokinetic properties. It has successfully been used in combination with subtherapeutic doses of CSA to treat a woman with severe psoriasis refractory to traditional therapies.[2] However, long-term and large-scale studies are needed to establish the efficacy and safety of everolimus in psoriasis.

Note: CSA—Cyclosporine.

REFERENCES

1. Reitamo S, Spuls P, Sassolas B, Lahfa M, Claudy A, Griffiths CE. Sirolimus European Psoriasis Study Group. Efficacy of sirolimus (rapamycin) administered concomitantly with a subtherapeutic dose of cyclosporin in the treatment of severe psoriasis: A randomized controlled trial. Br J Dermatol. 2001;145:438-45.
2. Frigerio E, Colombo MD, Franchi C, Altomare A, Garutti C, Altomare GF. Severe psoriasis treated with a new macrolide: Everolimus. Br J Dermatol. 2007;156:372-4.

Chapter

32

Thiazolidinediones in Psoriasis

Thiazolidinediones (TZD) are hypoglycemic agents and are used as insulin sensitizers in type 2 diabetes mellitus. These drugs are believed to lower insulin resistance in peripheral tissues and reduce hepatic glucose output by binding to peroxisome proliferator-activated receptor (PPAR) gamma. In a double-blind, randomized, placebo-controlled study to test the efficacy of pioglitazone in psoriasis, seventy patients with moderate to severe psoriasis received either pioglitazone 15 mg or pioglitazone 30 mg or placebo for 10 weeks. The percentage reduction in mean PASI scores was 21.6, 41.1 and 47.5% in the placebo, pioglitazone 15 m and 30 mg groups, respectively (thus higher dose was noted to be more effective). Pioglitazone was noted to be remarkably safe, with the exception of fall in hemoglobin in one patient and elevation of liver enzymes in two patients (Shafiq et al.).[1] Pioglitazone has been reported to be effective in psoriatic arthritis also (Bongartz et al.) and has been used in combination with retinoids especially acitretin with synergistic benefits. Psoriasis with metabolic syndrome is believed to be the main indication for the use of pioglitazone as it is an insulin sensitizer. It is suggested that it may help the psoriasis patients to fight the metabolic dysfunction, including insulin resistance, obesity, dyslipidemia and cardiovascular diseases, which is showing a greater association with psoriasis with each passing day.[2,3]

REFERENCES

1. Shafiq N, Malhotra S, Pandhi P, Gupta M, Kumar B, Sandhu K. Pilot trial: Pioglitazone versus placebo in patients with plaque psoriasis (the P6). Int J Dermatol. 2005;44:328-33.
2. Mittal R, Malhotra S, Pandhi P, Kaur I, Dogra S. Efficacy and safety of combination Acitretin and Pioglitazone therapy in patients with moderate to severe chronic plaque-type psoriasis: A randomized, double-blind, placebo-controlled clinical trial. Arch Dermatol. 2009;145:387-93.
3. Bongartz T, Coras B, Vogt T, Schφlmerich J, Móller-Ladner U. Treatment of active psoriatic arthritis with the PPARgamma ligand pioglitazone: An open-label pilot study. Rheumatology (Oxford). 2005;44:126-9.

Chapter

33

Paclitaxel in Psoriasis

Paclitaxel is a chemotherapeutic agent having antiproliferative, antiangiogenic and anti-inflammatory properties. In a phase-II pilot study involving 12 severe psoriatic patients, there was a dose-dependent response with decrease in PASI scores varying from 15% to 80% in different patients, who were put on paclitaxel. Two patients developed hypersensitivity reactions, whereas none developed myelosuppression.[1]

Nanoemulsion formulation of paclitaxel has been suggested to enhance the oral bioavailability of the drug in rats. However, these newer formulations need evaluation in humans and psoriatic patients to establish their efficacy and safety.[2]

REFERENCES

1. Ehrlich A, Booher S, Becerra Y, Borris DL, Figg WD, Turner ML, et al. Micellar paclitaxel improves severe psoriasis in a prospective phase II pilot study. J Am Acad Dermatol. 2004;50:533-40.
2. Khandavilli S, Panchagnula R. Nanoemulsions as versatile formulations for paclitaxel delivery: peroral and dermal delivery studies in rats. J Invest Dermatol. 2007;127:154-62.

Chapter

34 Neovastat in Psoriasis

The antiangiogenic agent neovastat is a new therapeutic approach in the management of psoriasis but more extensive studies need to be done before the drug is approved for the treatment of psoriasis. Neovastat (AE-941), is extracted from shark cartilage by homogenization and ultrafiltration. It is a vascular endothelial growth factor (VEGF) antagonist and has been shown to have antiangiogenic and anti-inflammatory properties in an in vitro assay.[1] In a randomized phase I/II dose-comparison clinical trial which involved 49 psoriasis patients, who were prescribed 60 mL, 120 mL, and 240 mL/day of neovastat, a statistically significant decrease in PASI score in 30.8%, 41.7% and 50% of the patients was noted (Sauder et al.). Nausea, vomiting, diarrhea, flatulence and constipation, acne and skin rash were the predominant side effects.[2]

REFERENCES

1. Dupont E, Savard PE, Jourdain C, Juneau C, Thibodeau A, Ross N, et al. Antiangiogenic properties of a novel shark cartilage extract: potential role in the treatment of psoriasis. J Cutan Med Surg. 1998;2:146-52.
2. Sauder DN, Dekoven J, Champagne P, Croteau D, Dupont E. Neovastat (AE-941), an inhibitor of angiogenesis: Randomized phase I/II clinical trial results in patients with plaque psoriasis. J Am Acad Dermatol. 2002;47: 535-41.

Chapter 35 The Strength of Recommendations for the Treatment of Psoriasis Using Traditional Systemic Therapies

Practising evidence-based medicine is dependent on finding and utilizing the best evidence. An important principle of evidence-based medicine is that the quality (strength) of evidence is based on a hierarchy of evidence. The hierarchy of evidence consists of results of well-designed experimental studies, such as RCTs (randomized controlled studies), results of observational studies, such as case series, expert opinion and personal experience in descending order.

The strength of recommendations of various systemic therapies for psoriasis is summarized in Table 35.1.

TABLE 35.1: The strength of recommendations for the treatment of psoriasis using traditional systemic therapies

Agent	Strength of recommendation	Level of evidence
Methotrexate	B	II
Cyclosporine	B	II
Acitretin	B	II
Azathioprine	C	III
Fumaric acid esters	B	I
Hydroxyurea	C	III
Leflunomide	B	II
Mycophenolate mofetil	C	III
Sulfasalazine	B	II
Tacrolimus	B	II
6-Thioguanine	C	III

WHAT DO YOU MEAN BY LEVEL OF EVIDENCE OF A STUDY? (TABLE 35.2)

TABLE 35.2: Level of evidence of various types of studies

Level of evidence	Type of study
1a.	Multiple RCTs with homogeneity
1b.	Individual RCT (with narrow confidence interval)

Contd...

Contd...

Level of evidence	Type of study
1c.	All or none (Interventions that produced dramatic increase in survival or outcome, such as streptomycin for tuberculous meningitis)
2a.	Cohort studies with homogeneity
2b.	Individual cohort study (including low-quality RCT, e.g. <80% follow-up)
2c.	Outcomes research (includes cost-benefit,cost-effectiveness and cost-utility analyses)
3a.	Case-control studies with homogeneity
3b.	Individual case-control study
4.	Case series (poor-quality cohort and case-control studies)
5.	Expert opinion without explicit critical appraisal, or based on physiology, bench research or logical deduction

WHAT ARE THE GRADES OF RECOMMENDATION?

A. Recommendation based on consistent and good-quality patient-oriented evidence.
B. Recommendation based on inconsistent and limited-quality patient-oriented evidence.
C. Recommendation based on consensus, opinion, or case studies.

SUGGESTED READING

1. McCarthy CM, Collins ED, Pusic AL. Where do we find the best evidence? Plast Reconstr Surg. 2008;122: 1942-7.
2. Chung KC, Ram AN. Evidence-based medicine: the fourth revolution in American medicine? Plast Reconstr Surg. 2009;123:389-98.

Chapter 36

Investigational Therapies in Psoriasis

The various investigational therapies for psoriasis are summarized below.

JANUS KINASE INHIBITORS

Tofacitinib is a drug of the Janus kinase (JAK) inhibitor class. It is currently approved for the treatment of rheumatoid arthritis in the United States and is being studied for the treatment of psoriasis, inflammatory bowel disease and other immunological diseases, as well as for the prevention of organ-transplant rejection.

IMMUNOTHERAPY

Most of the treatment modalities in psoriasis provide only symptomatic relief and do not lead to permanent cure or long-term remission. Immunotherapy is under evaluation so as to produce immunomodulation and long-term remission. Immunotherapy probably works by inducing a transient Th1 response with compensatory Th2 response. After preliminary investigations, two intradermal injections of heat-killed suspension of *Mycobacterium vaccae* (*M. vaccae*) were given at 3 weeks interval to chronic plaque psoriatic patients. Improvement in PASI score was seen in 19 of 21 patients and the improvement persisted for 6 months. A subsequent study supported its efficacy.

Balagon et al. tested psoriasis vaccine (PVAC) which is a more potent derivative of *M. vaccae*. It contains heat-killed, delipidated, deglycolipidated *M. vaccae*. In an open trial, 65% patients showed more than 50% reduction in the PASI score at 12 weeks after the injections. In two subsequent studies investigating PVAC in psoriasis and psoriatic arthritis (PsA) patients, it was found to be ineffective.

Mw (Mycobacterium w) vaccine has been tried in psoriatic patients in small studies. Rath et al. conducted a pilot study in which 24 patients received two injections of Mw vaccine at 3 weeks interval. In 4 months, 16.6% had marked improvement (>50% reduction in PASI), 62.5% had moderate improvement (25–50% reduction in PASI) and 16.6% showed no change (<25% reduction). Subsequently, this vaccine was tested in 45 patients with mild to moderate plaque-type psoriasis. In this study,the results were not encouraging, with less than 40% patients showing mild to moderate improvement.

Another vaccine, psoraxine, which was originally developed to induce resistance against leishmaniasis, is still in experimental stages for psoriasis.

REFERENCES

1. Lehrer A, Bressanelli A, Wachsmann V, Bottasso O, Bay ML, Singh M, et al. Immunotherapy with *Mycobacterium vaccae* in the treatment of psoriasis. FEMS Immunol Med Microbiol. 1998;21:71-7.

TYROSINE KINASE INHIBITORS

There are individual reports of clinical improvement in psoriasis with tyrosine kinase inhibitors (TKI) when given to cancer patients. SU-011248 is a VEGF receptor-tyrosine kinase inhibitor which has been tried in psoriasis. Further prospective randomized control studies however, need to be done to prove their efficacy.[1,2]

REFERENCES

1. Wierzbicka E, Tourani JM, Guillet G. Improvement of psoriasis and cutaneous side-effects during tyrosine kinase inhibitor therapy for renal metastatic adenocarcinoma. A role for epidermal growth factor receptor (EGFR) inhibitors in psoriasis? Br J Dermatol. 2006;155:213-4.
2. Keshtgarpour M, Dudek. AZ SU-011248, a vascular endothelial growth factor receptor-tyrosine kinase inhibitor, controls chronic psoriasis. Transl Res. 2007;149:103-6.

PHOSPHODIESTERASES

The phosphodiesterases (PDE) are the enzymes which degrade second messenger molecules cAMP and cGMP. They have broad anti-inflammatory effects and therefore have been tried in psoriasis and atopic dermatitis. Dose-limiting side effects of PDEs are nausea, diarrhea, vomiting and abdominal pain. In a pilot study, oral apremilast, a PDE-4 inhibitor, was given to 19 psoriatic patients. There was improvement in 73% of cases with mild adverse effects. Long-term studies are however needed.[1]

REFERENCES

1. Gottlieb AB, Strober B, Krueger JG, Rohane P, Zeldis JB, Hu CC, et al. An open-label, single-arm pilot study in patients with severe plaque-type psoriasis treated with an oral anti-inflammatory agent, apremilast. Curr Med Res Opin. 2008;24:1529-38.

CHEMOKINE RECEPTOR BLOCKERS

SCH527123 (Schering Plough) is an allosteric antagonist of CXCR1 and CXCR2 which inhibits neutrophil chemotaxis and release of myeloperoxidase in response to CXCL8 and CXCL1. These are in experimental stages.

PEPTIDE-T IN PSORIASIS

Peptide-T is a synthetic octapeptide that shares a segment of the envelope glycoprotein (gp 120) of the HIV. Its use in an HIV-negative patient of psoriasis with PA was reported for the first time in 1989.It is speculated that peptide-T acts by inhibition of interferon (IFN)-gamma production and induction of interleukin (IL)-10. Marcusson et al. treated nine patients of recalcitrant and long-standing psoriasis with 2 mg peptide-T intravenous daily injections given for 28 days. Eight of them showed less than 50% improvement by day 28 and five patients had more than 50% improvement at 3 months. Limitations with peptides are that they exhibit poor absorption, get easily metabolized and are immunogenic.[1-3]

REFERENCES

1. Marcusson JA, Wetterberg L. Peptide-T in the treatment of psoriasis and psoriatic arthritis. A case report. Acta Derm Venereol. 1989;69:86-8.
2. Raychaudhuri SP, Farber EM, Raychaudhuri SK. Immunomodulatory effects of peptide T on Th 1/Th 2 cytokines. Int J Immunopharmacol. 1999;21:609-15.
3. Marcusson JA, Talme T, Wetterberg L, Johansson O. Peptide T a new treatment for psoriasis? A study of nine patients. Acta Derm Venereol. 1991;71:479-83.

p38 MITOGEN-ACTIVATED PROTEIN KINASE INHIBITOR

Intracellular protein cascades, such as mitogen-activated protein kinases (MAPK) are involved in cell cycle kinetics. Novel p38 MAPK inhibitor, BMS-582949, is in phase-II studies for inflammatory diseases including rheumatoid arthritis, psoriasis and atherosclerosis.[1]

REFERENCES

1. Norman P. BMS-582949: crystalline form of a p38 alpha inhibitor? WO2008079857. Expert Opin Ther Pat. 2009;19:1165-8.

PROTEIN KINASE C INHIBITORS

Protein kinase C (PKC) inhibitors block early T cell activation. AEB071, a PKC inhibitor strongly and selectively inhibits the classical (a, b) and the novel theta (q)-PKC isoforms. In a recently published study, AEB071 was given orally to 32 patients with severe plaque psoriasis for 2 weeks. There was a dose-dependent response, with PASI 75 achieved in 69% of the treatment group receiving 300 mg twice daily. Larger patient cohorts and longer treatment periods are required to establish its safety and efficacy in psoriasis.[1]

REFERENCES

1. Skvara H, Dawid M, Kleyn E, Wolff B, Meingassner JG, Knight H, et al. The PKC inhibitor AEB071 may be a therapeutic option for psoriasis. J Clin Invest. 2008;118:3151-9.

NERVE GROWTH FACTOR RECEPTOR BLOCKER

The use of nerve growth factor (NGF) receptor blocker is an experimental therapy for psoriasis and at an infancy stage presently. Recent research supports the role of NGFs and neurogenic inflammation in the pathogenesis of psoriasis. Novel therapeutic agent K252a is a high-affinity NGF receptor blocker. It has been reported to improve psoriatic plaques in severe combined immunodeficient mouse-human skin model of psoriasis.[1,2]

REFERENCES

1. Raychaudhuri SP, Raychaudhuri SK. Role of NGF and neurogenic inflammation in the pathogenesis of psoriasis. Prog Brain Res. 2004;146:433-7.
2. Raychaudhuri SP, Sanyal M, Weltman H, Kundu-Raychaudhuri S. K252a, a high-affinity nerve growth factor receptor blocker, improves psoriasis: An in vivo study using the severe combined immunodeficient mouse-human skin model. J Invest Dermatol. 2004;122:812-9.

CONCLUSION

Treatment of psoriasis is still evolving. Methotrexate, cyclosporine and retinoids are well-established and time-tested drugs. In recent times, there has been a vast expansion in the armamentarium of therapeutic agents for psoriasis with the entry of exciting new era of biologic therapy. Long-term experience with biologics is still limited, both with regard to efficacy and, more importantly, safety. Although preliminary results are encouraging, these drugs are also not curative, need parenteral administration, have significant adverse effects and additionally, loss of efficacy on long-term therapy as well as disease unresponsiveness have been observed. Therefore, the search for safer, orally-administered newer and cheaper drugs is imperative.

SUGGESTED READINGS

1. Bansback N, Sizto S, Sun H, et al. Efficacy of systemic treatments for moderate to severe plaque psoriasis: Systematic review and meta-analysis. Dermatology. 2009;219(3):209-18.

Chapter

37 Phototherapy in Psoriasis

Phototherapy deals with the use of nonionising electromagnetic radiation to bring about a beneficial effect on a particular disease. Photochemotherapy refers to a similar effect brought about by UV radiation when used in combination with chemicals like psoralens. Before the advent of modern scientific thought, sunlight was used for its beneficial effect by the ancient Indian and Egyptian civilizations thousands of years back. Niels Finsen first used UV light from a carbon arc lamp to treat lupus vulgaris in 1890 which heralded the era of modern phototherapy. El Mofty in 1948 and later Lerner et al. studied the response of vitiligo to topical and oral psoralens. The term PUVA was coined for the use of psoralen and UVA in the treatment of psoriasis. In recent years the use of psoralen bath has become popular. Bath PUVA originated in Scandinavia. During the past decade, new devices and developments in phototherapy has opened new avenues for the treatment of photoresponsive dermatoses. The development of narrow-band UVB and high-dose UV-A1 has broadened the clinical spectrum of diseases that can be treated with phototherapy.[1,2]

PUVA (psoralens with UVA) is an established therapy for psoriasis. There is, however, increasing concern about the long-term safety of PUVA because of the now well-documented increased risk of nonmelanoma skin cancer and, more recently, reported risk of melanoma. Studies of wavelength-dependence of the response of psoriasis to UVB (290–320 nm) phototherapy have led to the development of the TL-01 fluorescent UVB lamps in which 83% of the UV emission is at 311 ± 2 nm, a spectral region known to be effective at clearing psoriasis. The development of the TL-O1 lamp with higher therapeutic potential than broad-band UVB source and less carcinogenic risk than PUVA has led to the continuously growing use of NBUVB therapy in psoriasis.

Although PUVA therapy of psoriasis is clearly more effective than conventional broad-band phototherapy, there are few studies available comparing PUVA with the new modality of NBUVB phototherapy. These studies have suggested that NBUVB may have therapeutic efficacy equal to PUVA and at the same time is associated with less adverse effects.[3]

UVA Phototherapy*:* UVA ranges from 320–400 nm and constitutes 90–95% of UVR reaching earth's surface. It is divided into UVA-II (32–340 nm) and UVA-1 (340–400 nm). UVA is known to penetrate beyond dermis and result in tanning of skin, erythema and burn which is maximum after 72 hours. It is least influenced by atmosphere and geographical factors. UVA is carcinogenic and causes ageing of the skin.[4]

UV-B phototherapy*:* Ultraviolet B rays constitute 5–10% of the ultraviolet radiation reaching earth's surface. They range from 280 to 320 nm. They penetrate the epidermis and are potent and harmful. UVB produces erythema and indirect tanning. It is influenced to a great extent by atmosphere and geographical factors (Figs 37.1 and 37.2).[5]

Goeckerman and Ingrams regimen use the UVB component of UV light in treatment of psoriasis. UVB acts by damaging DNA, RNA and cell membrane by induction of photoproducts. With the development of UVB-narrow band fluorescent lamps by Philips (Philips TL-01) the prospects of better treatment for psoriasis has brightened. The TL-01 emits UV light at 311 nm which matches the therapeutic optimum for faster clearance and longer remission in psoriasis. The duration of treatment is reduced to 1/3rd that of PUVA and broad-band UVB. Comparative studies have demonstrated that NBUVB 311nm and PUVA are equally effective. Carcinogenic effect of UVB 311nm is reduced significantly due to the decreased duration of treatment and it is cost effective compared to PUVA. Combinations include giving NB-UVB with dithranol, etretinate, tazarotene and PUVA. Retinoids have a beneficial effect on psoriasis and in addition have anticarcinogenic property which further reduces the risk of UVB-induced skin malignancies.[6]

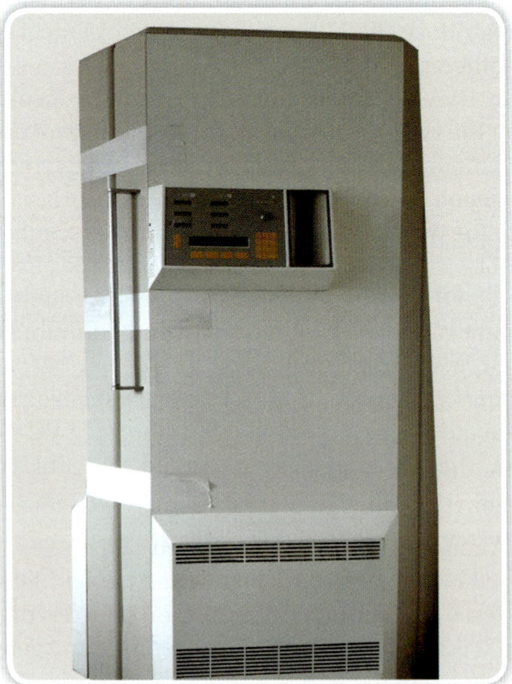

FIG. 37.1: Whole-body UVA and UVB phototherapy chamber with display panel

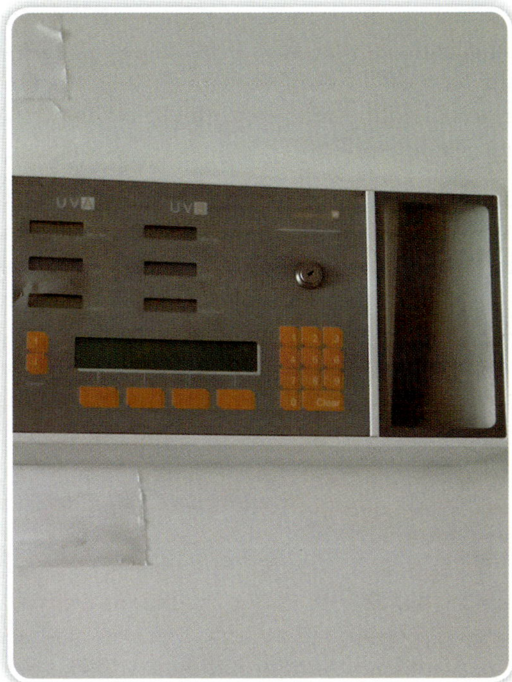

FIG. 37.2: Display panel of whole-body UVA and UVB phototherapy chamber

High-dose UVA-1 Phototherapy: Another advance in the field of phototherapy has been the use of high-dose UVA-1 (340–400 nm) light. This can be used as a monotherapy in several inflammatory skin disorders. It is most useful in the treatment of atopic dermatitis. The dose given is as high as 130 J/cm^2 daily for 15 consecutive days. The long-term risks of UVA-1 are yet to be evaluated, hence it is not recommended in persons below 18 years of age. Clinical scoring system and monitoring of eosinophilic cationic protein (ECP) was used in assessing its therapeutic efficacy. Urticaria pigmentosa and localized scleroderma are the other conditions in which high-dose UVA-1 has been tried. High-dose UVA-1 needs a special light source.[7]

Photodynamic therapy: Photodynamic therapy (PDT) is the treatment of skin diseases by generating highly-reactive oxygen intermediates by interaction of light with photosensitizers. PDT uses longer-wavelength blue light with deeper penetration to generate oxygen intermediates. The photosensitizing drugs used for dermatologic conditions are porphyrins, 5aminolevulinic acid (ALA) and benzo porphyrin derivatives. Free radicals produced cause cell damage. PDT is used for treating basal cell carcinoma (BCC), squamous cell carcinoma (SCC), cutaneous T cell lymphomas (CTCL) and, kaposi's sarcoma. Among the nonmalignant conditions psoriasis, genital warts and actinic keratoses have been reported to respond to PDT. Preferential localization of the drug in tumor cells, because of its difference in vasculature makes it more useful in such diseases. PDT drugs are excited by UV light to triplet state. These excited drugs form free radicals and transfer energy to molecular oxygen to form singlet oxygen, which destroys abnormal cells.[8]

Photopheresis: It is used in advanced cases of CTCL and involves the ex vivo exposure of peripheral white blood cells to 8-MOP and UVA, which is followed by reinfusion to the circulation. Because of the decreased risk of side effects than that of conventional PUVA this treatment has been suggested in dermatological conditions like psoriasis, scleroderma, atopic dermatitis, pemphigus and SLE. However, its practical use remains minimal.[9]

Phototherapy in psoriasis with HIV infection: This is a controversial issue as both phototherapy and photochemotherapy can induce suppression of immunity which can lead to worsening of HIV status. It has been suggested that viral gene transcription and virus production could get a boost as the HIV promoter gets activated. It is also reported that HIV-induced immune suppression could accelerate skin carcinomas due to UV radiation. On the other hand several reports point to the beneficial effects UVB and PUVA have on pruritus and psoriasis that manifest in HIV infection. However, long-term observations are required to come to an appropriate conclusion. The available data suggest that UVB is more likely to be harmful than PUVA in HIV-infected persons.[10]

PHOTOCHEMOTHERAPY

Photochemotherapy refers to the use of PUVA (psoralens with UVA) in photoresponsive dermatoses. The basis of PUVA is to induce remission of skin diseases by repeated controlled phototoxic reactions, when psoralens are activated by UVA. The exact mechanism of action of psoralens is not fully understood, but they mainly produce their actions by two types of reactions. Type 1 is oxygen independent which results in formation of mono and bi-functional adducts (due to interaction of psoralens with cellular nucleotides) which inhibit DNA synthesis. The type 2 reaction is oxygen dependent resulting in oxidation of cellular contents leading to cell damage. Psoralens with UVA is also known to suppress abnormal immune response and kill inflammatory cells. In vitiligo, PUVA therapy stimulates melanogenesis by photoconjunction to DNA in melanocytes resulting in increased proliferation and distribution of the cells. It also stimulates production of larger melanosomes and their transfer to keratinocytes. Tyrosine synthesis is also stimulated. Certain precautionary measures need to be followed with PUVA therapy which includes the use of UVA-blocking glasses during and 24 hours after treatment, broad-spectrum sunscreens and protective genital shield in males.[11]

PUVASOL

Psoralens with sunlight as the source of ultraviolet A-rays is known as PUVASOL. In centers where artificial chambers are not available, PUVASOL is the most commonly used mode of treatment. Here both UVA and UVB in sunlight result in photoaugmentation and photoaddition. A major disadvantage of solar irradiation as a light source is the difficulty in quantifying UV light, as the total amount of UVA reaching the skin at any one time varies widely depending on the season, time of the day, latitude and conditions of the atmosphere. Other disadvantages are lack of privacy, difficulty in monitoring the dose of ultraviolet rays and in addition to ultraviolet A, ultraviolet B, infrared rays and visible light which are not needed for PUVA therapy may lead to undesirable side effects. UVB in sunlight can increase the thickness of epidermis and this makes the sun-exposed skin leathery and this may interfere with the effectiveness. The main advantages of sunlight as a source of PUVA is that it is inexpensive and patients need not travel long distance for treatment.[12]

Topical Treatment

The application of methoxypsoralen (8-MOP) in creams, ointments or lotions followed by UVA irradiation is effective in limited-plaque psoriasis and for palmoplantar disease. It can also be used to induce repigmentation over streaks of residual depigmentation following punch grafting and when other measures fail to induce pigmentation.

Methodology

A lotion containing 0.1–1% 8-MOP is applied and exposed to sunlight either immediately or after one to two hours. This treatment is given three to four times weekly with UVA dose being gradually increased. Maintenance dose may be needed. Among the psoralens, trimethyl psoralen (TMP) is most convenient for topical application because of its weak penetrability. The penetrated drug makes photo adducts with DNA molecules even if UVA light is given as soon as the drug is painted resulting in significant inhibition of epidermal DNA synthesis. The advantages of topical psoralen therapy are that systemic side effects can be avoided. The disadvantages are that topical PUVA is laborious and time-consuming, as every lesion has to be treated individually. The formation of erythema and blisters is more common with topical psoralen application and intense irregular pigmentation may be seen at the site of treated plaques.[13]

Bathwater Delivery of 8-MOP and Trioxsalen

Bathwater psoralen delivery plus UVA has also been found to be equal to or better than local application of psoralen with ointments, creams or lotions. Psoralen bathwater delivery eliminates the laborious application required with other topical modalities. The even skin distribution delivered by bathwater leads to even pigmentation. Bathwater delivery of 8-MOP has been found to be as effective as oral administration of 8-MOP and requires smaller amounts of UVA radiation and is associated with fewer side effects.

Methodology

The psoralen bathwater solutions are prepared by diluting 50 mL of 8-MOP in 100 liters of water resulting in a final concentration of 3.75 mg/L. The patients are made to soak for 15 minutes in this solution and then quickly wipe dry. Subsequently the patients are given whole-body irradiation with UVA. The initial dose depending upon the skin type.[14]

Bath-suit Delivery of Psoralen

Bath-suit therapy is another modality found to be an effective therapy for psoriasis. Advantages of bath-suit delivery of 8-MOP are that it requires only two liters of water and 0.8 mL of 8-MOP solution when compared to bathwater therapy which needs 100 liters of water and 50 mL of 8-MOP. The cost of the drug is less and it is easy and less time-consuming with no systemic side effects when compared to oral and topical psoralen therapy. This treatment can be carried out at home with sunlight as the UVA source. The disadvantages of bath-suit delivery are that the entire body surface especially face does not come in contact with the drug and the concentration of the drug may not be uniform in the bath suit.[15]

PUVA Turban Therapy

This therapy has been used in the treatment of alopecia areata.

Methodology

A cotton towel is soaked with a 0.0001% 8-MOP solution in a dose of 1 mg/L at 37°C, wrung gently to remove excess water and wrapped around the patient's head in a turban fashion for 20 min. This is directly followed by UVA irradiation. Treatment sessions are three to four times per week. This therapy has been shown to be well tolerated and is an efficient therapeutic alternative in the treatment of alopecia areata.[16]

Oral Treatment

In oral PUVA therapy, 8-methoxypsoralen (8-MOP) is administered orally in a dose of 0.6–0.8 mg per kg body weight and 5-MOP in a dose of 1.2–1.8 mg per kilogram body weight 1–3 hours before light exposure, depending on the absorption characteristics of the particular drug.

The initial UVA doses are established by either skin typing (American protocol) or by minimal phototoxic dose (MPD) testing (European protocol). The MPD is defined as the minimal dose of UVA that produces a barely perceptible, but well-defined, erythema when photoprotected areas of the skin (e.g. bottocks, upper back) are exposed to increasing doses of UVA ranging from 0.5 to 5 J/cm. The erythema readings are performed 72 hours after testing, at which time the psoralen phototoxicity reaction usually reaches its peak. It is difficult to determine MPD in the Indian skin and therapy is usually started with an initial dose of 0.5 J/cm^2 and increments of 10–20% are then made every second or third sitting. The frequency of treatments is reduced after satisfactory clearing of disease and the last UVA dose is used as a maintenance dose if maintenance treatment is planned. The duration of this maintenance phase and the frequency of treatments depends on the particular disease being treated and its propensity to relapse. It is recommended to protect eyes with UVA-blocking glasses for 12–24 hours on the day of exposure. A sunscreen with an SPF of at least 15 is required for protection from a psoralen phototoxic reaction. Males should also shield their genitalia.[17]

Side Effects and Contraindications[18]

A. Short-term side effects: The short-term side effects of PUVA therapy are:

1. *Due to oral methoxypsoralen:* Gastrointestinal disturbances, CNS disturbances, drug fever, exanthems and hepatotoxicity.
2. *Phototoxic reactions:* Symptomatic erythema (most common, seen in 10% of cases), pruritis, photoonycholysis, Koebner's phenomenon, Friction blisters on hands and feet, hypertrichosis, phytophotodermatitis and subacute phototoxicity.
3. *Others:* Herpes simplex recurrences and photosensitive eruptions.

B. Long-term side effects: Photoageing, Melanoma and nonmelanoma skin cancer and anterior cortical cataracts.

Because PUVA therapy is based on photosensitizing effects, it is contraindicated in patients with photosensitive diseases, such as systemic lupus erythematosus and porphyria cutanea tarda. PUVA therapy is also contraindicated in pregnant women because of concerns about possible teratogenicity.

Protocols for PUVA:[19] There are various protocols for PUVA which are;

1. *US protocol:* American Academy of Dermatology recommends determining skin type before starting phototherapy. First-exposure dose is given based on skin typing and is given 2–3 times per week. Increments range from 0.5–1.5 J/cm^2 depending on the response.
2. *European protocol:* In this protocol, MPD has to be determined before giving the first dose. Four treatments are given per week on 2 consecutive days followed by a rest day and then next 2 daily doses (11 0 11). Increments are given only after the first week and range from 0.5 to 2 J/cm^2.
3. *Manipal protocol:* Studies done in Manipal have failed to demonstrate minimal phototoxicity dose (MPD) in Indian skin. In this protocol, a starting dose of 4–6J/cm^2 with increments of 0.5J/cm^2 depending on response is recommended. The maximum dose suggested is 18 J/cm^2. Treatment is given 3–4 times per week.

***Protocol for NB-UVB*:** Before starting NB-UVB, it is recommended to determine the minimal erythema dose (MED) first. Initially give 70% of MED, which is known as near MED. Far MED (35% MED) has also been used in some studies. Subsequently if no erythema occurs, increase the dose by 20%. If there is minimal erythema, maintain same dose. If there is well-defined erythema, postpone the therapy until next visit, give the same dose and later increase by only 10%. If there is painful erythema, edema or bullae, withhold treatment until recovery, then reduce exposure to half the starting dose and subsequently increase by 10% at each visit. End point of treatment is clearance of the disease.[20]

Note: Minimal erythema dose is the minimum dose of UV light that produces barely perceptible and well-defined erythema. MED testing is carried on covered sites, such as buttocks and read after 72 hours of light exposure. Ideally MED should be determined before the initiation of UVB therapy. Phototherapy is started with 50% of MED dose.

Points to Remember

- Lupus vulgaris is the disease in which light therapy was first tried
- NB-UVB has therapeutic efficacy equal to PUVA
- NB-UVB is likely to be devoid of side-effects and will be considerably safe in the long-term than PUVA
- MED or MPD should be determined prior to the use of NBUVB and PUVA
- PUVA can be combined with retinoids, methotrexate, UVB and topical tazarotene
- The Pregnancy category status of psoralens is C
- Calcipotriol should not be used concomitantly with phototheray as it gets degraded by phototherapy
- Salicylic acid has photoprotective properties which will reduce the efficacy of phototherapy, hence should not be used concomitantly with phototherapy.

Note: NB-UVB therapy—Narrow band Ultravoilet B light therapy; PUVA—Psoralen with UVA light therapy; MPD—Minimal phototoxicity dose; MED—Minimal erythema dose.

REFERENCES

1. Harber LC. PUVA therapy status. J Am Acad Dermatol. 1979;1:150-1.
2. Roenigk HH, Farber EM, Storrs F. Photochemotherapy for psoriasis. Arch Dermatol. 1979;115:576-9.
3. Hell E, Hodgson C, Manna V. Psoralen photochemotherapy of psoriasis. Br J Dermatol. 1979;101:293-8.
4. Farber EM, Abel EA, Cox AJ. Long-term risks of psoralen and UV-A therapy for psoriasis. Arch Dermatol. 1983; 119: 426-31.
5. Larko O, Swanbeck G. Is UVB therapy of psoriasis safe? Acta Derm Venereol. 1982;62:507-12.
6. Goeckerman WH. Treatment of psoriasis. Arch Dermatol Syphilol. 1931;24:446-50.
7. Adrian RM, Parrish JA, Momtas TK, et al. Outpatient phototherapy for psoriasis. Arch Dermatol. 1981;117: 623-6.
8. Honigsmann H, Szeimies RM, Knobler R, et al. Photochemotherapy and Photodynamic Therapy, In: Dermatology in General Medicine, 5h Edn, Edited by Fitzpatrick et al, McGraw Hill Book Company, New York. 1999;2880-900.
9. Lord JT, Ziboth VA, Poitier J. The effects of photosensitisers and UV irradiation on the biosynthesis and metabolism of prostaglandins. Br J Dermatol. 1976;95:397-406.
10. McEvoy MT, Stern RS. Psoralens and related compounds in the treatment of psoriasis. Pharmacol Ther. 1987;34:75-97.
11. Lowe NJ, Weingarten D, Bourget T, et al. PUVA therapy for psoriasis: comparison of oral and bath-water delivery of 8-methoxypsoralen. J Am Acad Dermatol. 1986;14:754-60.
12. Marquis L, Rangwala GM. Photochemotherapy of psoriasis with oral 8-MOP and solarirradiation (PUVASOL) therapy.Indian J Dermatol Venereol Leprol. 1980;46:287-93.
13. Schaefer H, Vivell K, Kentesch V. Simplification of topical therapy for psoriasis with 8-MOP: methods and initial results. Br J Dermatol. 1976;94:363-7.
14. Fischer T. Advantages of bath PUVA. Seminar Dermatol. 1985;4:297-9.
15. Hannuksela M, Karvonen J. Trioxsalen bath plus UVA is effective and safe in the treatment of psoriasis. Br J Dermatol. 1987;99:703-7.
16. Dano K, Horio T, Ozaki M. Topical 8-methoxypsoralen photochemotherapy of psoriasis. Br J Dermatol. 1983;108: 519-24.
17. Melksi J, Tanenbaum L, Parrish JA, et al. Oral methoxsalen photochemotherapy for treatment of psoriasis; a cooperative clinical trial. J Invest Dermatol. 1977;68:328-35.
18. Stern RS, Thibodeau LA, Kleinerman RA, et al. Risk of cutaneous carcinoma in patients treated with oral methoxsalen photochemotherapy for psoriasis. N Eng J Med. 1979;300:809-13.
19. Reusch M, Christophers E. Psoriasis: a continuing challenge for phototherapy. Curr Prob Dermatol. 1986;15:219-31.
20. Green C, Ferguson J, Lakshmipathi T, Johnson BE. 311 nm UVB phototherapy: an effective treatment for psoriasis. Br J Dermatol. 1988;119:691-6.

Chapter

38

Recent Advances in Phototherapy

Phototherapy is a bridging link in the treatment of psoriasis between topical and systemic anti-psoriatic therapies. It is more effective than topical modalities and devoid of the toxic effects of systemic therapies. Phototherapy has undergone a sea change since its initial use in lupus vulgaris. Some of the recent advances in phototherapy are as follows:

1. Sublingual delivery of psoralens in skin type 1 and 2 is under research and is suggested to be useful. It may reduce the risk of hepatic and renal damage in patients who already have dysfunction of these two organs. Side effects like nausea and intolerance will also be reduced.
2. Bath PUVA wherein a patient immerses himself in a solution of psoralen before UVA exposure has been popular for quite sometime now. It has been found that it is much safer and better than other modalities of UV treatment in psoriasis.
3. Photodynamic therapy which is used for the treatment of actinic keratosis, BCC and other skin tumors has been found to be useful in psoriasis also.
4. Polyphenols present in green tea have a protective effect against skin damage caused by PUVA.
5. KUVA therapy: Khellin a furochomarin, derived from the plant ammi visnaga, which is known for its pigmentary properties was initially used as a coronary vasodilator. Oral khellin plus UVA (KUVA) has been used in the treatment of vitiligo since a long time. Given in a dose of 50–100 mg, 2.5 hours before UVA exposure, it produces significant repigmentation of vitiligo skin. It is less phototoxic and does not induce hyperpigmentation of nonvitiliginous skin.
6. BIOSKIN, a new device which can produce a focused beam of UVB has shown promise in the treatment of resistant cases of segmental vitiligo.[1,2]
7. NBUVB phototherapy, is a potential advance in UVB-based phototherapy and is increasingly being used in the treatment of psoriasis. However, only sparse data is available with regard to the relative therapeutic effectiveness of NBUVB and PUVA, and most of these earlier studies have compared these two modalities using half-body comparison. All these studies comparing NBUVB and PUVA are of the opinion that the clearance of psoriasis is faster with fewer number of treatments and days to clear in significantly greater proportion of patients using PUVA as compared to NBUVB, but the cumulative clearance dose for the NBUVB is significantly lower than PUVA (Gordan et al.). Markham et al. in an open, randomized and controlled study of 54 chronic plaque psoriatics treated with an equierythemogenic dosage of either thrice-weekly TL-O1 NBUVB or twice-weekly 8-MOP PUVA until completely clear, concluded that patients in the PUVA group required significantly fewer treatments than patients in the NBUVB group. However, they also showed that there was no statistically significant difference in the number of days to clear the psoriasis between the

TABLE 38.1: Comparison of UVA with UVB

UVA	UVB
It requires psoralens	It does not require psoralens
It is contraindicated in children <12 years of age, elderly patients, during pregnancy and lactation and in patients with compromised hepatic and renal functions	It can be given in children <12 years of age, elderly patients, during pregnancy and lactation and in patients with compromised hepatic and renal functions
Response is earlier with UVA	Response is sustained
Skin and eye protection against sunlight throughtout the day is required	No eye protection is required outside the chamber
Longer exposure time	Shorter exposure time
Side effects of psoralens	No side effects associated with psoralens
Less expensive	More expensive
More carcinogenic	Less carcinogenic

two groups. Adverse effects like grade-I erythema developed in all patients in both groups, indicating that both treatment modalities are erythemogenic. But, grade-II erythema and other adverse effects like nausea, vertigo, headache, pruritus and diffuse hair loss was observed more commonly in the PUVA group. Markham and Collins, have also reported fewer side-effects with NBUVB (TL-01) as compared to PUVA in an audit of adverse effects of oral 8MOP PUVA and NBUVB (TL-0l) in the management of chronic plaque psoriasis. Thus both NBUVB and PUVA are effective in the treatment of psoriasis, but patients in the PUVA group achieve faster clearance, require significantly fewer number of treatment sessions and fewer number of days to clear as compared to the NBUVB group. However, the mean cumulative clearance dose and adverse effects are lower in the NBUVB group than in the PUVA group (Table 38.1).[3,4,5]

Points to Remember

NBUVB phototherapy, is a potential advance in UVB-based phototherapy and is increasingly being used in the treatment of psoriasis. With regards to the relative therapeutic effectiveness of NBUVB and PUVA, however, only sparse data is available. The mean cumulative clearance dose and adverse effects are lower in the NBUVB group than in the PUVA group.

Note: NBUVB—Narrowband UVB; PUVA—Psoralen with UVA; 8-MOP—8-Methoxypsoralen.

REFERENCES

1. Van Weelden H, Young E, Van der Leun JC. Therapy of psoriasis: Comparison of photochemotherapy and several variants of phototherapy. Br J Dermatol. 1980;103:1-9.
2. Parrish JA, Jaenicke KF. Action spectrum for phototherapy of psoriasis. J Invest Dermatol. 1981;76:359-62.
3. Gadgil RB, Talwalkar PG. Photochemotherapy of psoriasis. Indian J Dermatol Venereol Leprol. 1980;46:294-8.
4. Dawe RS, Cameron H, Yule S. A randomized controlled trial of narrowband ultraviolet B vs bath-psoralen plus ultraviolet A photochemotherapy for psoriasis. Br J Dermatol. 2003;148:1194-204.
5. Momtaz K, Parrish JA JA. Combination of psoralens and ultraviolet A and ultraviolet B in the treatment of psoriasis vulgaris: a bilateral comparison study. J Am Acad Dermatol. 1984;10:481-6.

Chapter

39

Narrowband Ultraviolet B Phototherapy in the Treatment of Psoriasis

Ultraviolet (UV) light comprises a narrowband in the electromagnetic spectrum consisting of wavelengths between100 nm and 400 nm (UVC: 200–280 nm; UVB: 280–320 nm and UVA: 320–400 nm). UV light of shorter wavelengths is absorbed in the earth's atmosphere and only UV of longer wavelengths (UVA, UVB and minimal amount of UVC) reach the earth's surface. UV spectrum in the sunlight has been known to cure dermatological as well systemic diseases for ages. However, narrowband UVB (NBUVB) is a relatively recent but efficient introduction into dermatologic practice.[1]

UVB in combination with coal tar preparations is one of the oldest treatments for psoriasis. The Goekerman regimen introduced in 1925 comprises of UVB in addition to crude coal tar, an antimitotic agent and a photosensitizer. Broadband UVB (BBUVB) was used for quite sometime in the management of psoriasis after it had been introduced in 1978 by Wiskeman.[2] However, it never gained popularity due to its erythemogenic potential and lesser efficacy. The breakthrough in the use of UVB came in 1977 when Fischer, while examining the efficacy of wavelengths from 254 to 405 nm for the treatment of psoriasis, noted that a narrowband of UVB at 313 nm wavelength is notably effective for clearance of disease, particularly at higher doses, without producing significant erythema. Parrish and Jaenicke[3] discovered that clearance of psoriatic lesions occurred at wavelengths between 296 and 313 nm, with a better response at a wavelength of 313 nm.These findings gave impetus for the development of artificial fluorescent lamp containing phosphor (TL-01) producing peak emission at a narrow band of 311 nm (±2 nm). This development ushered in the era of new phototherapeutic modality (NBUVB) and several studies on its use in psoriasis and various other dermatoses followed. The first clinical use of this commercially available fluorescent lamp dates back to 1988 when van Weelden et al.[4] and Green et al. used it in the treatment of psoriasis. Subsequently, it has been used in indications other than the one it was developed for; with vitiligo, atopic eczema and mycosis fungoides being the more common ones (Figs 39.1 to 39.3).[2,3]

MECHANISM OF ACTION OF NB-UVB

The exact mechanism of action of NBUVB is not known. Following are the proposed mechanisms of NBUVB in psoriasis:[5]

1. NBUVB is known to cause the induction of several genetic and molecular factors.The most significant molecular target of NBUVB is cellular DNA. Absorption of UVB by nucleotides of nuclear DNA leads to DNA photoadduct or photoproduct formation, mainly pyrimidine dimers. These photoproducts interfere with cell cycle progression and induce growth

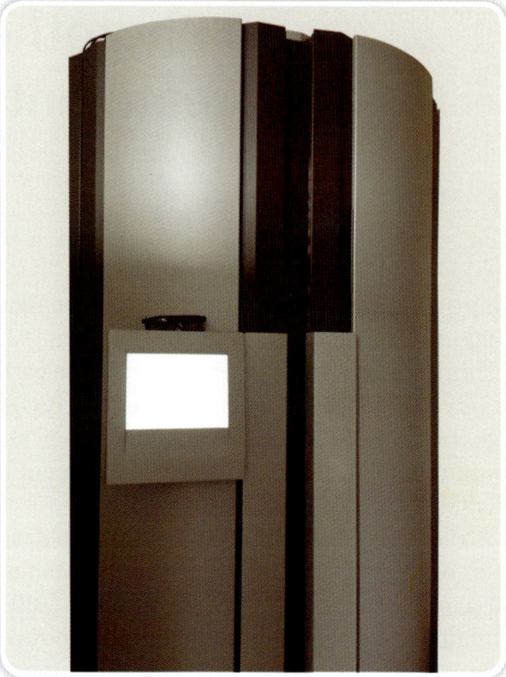

FIG. 39.1: Whole-body NB UVB chamber

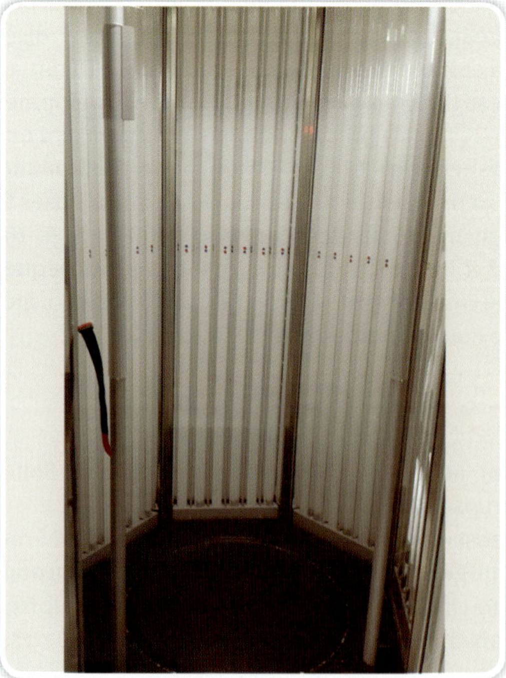

FIG. 39.2: Inside view of the NB UVB chamber showing fluorescent tube lights

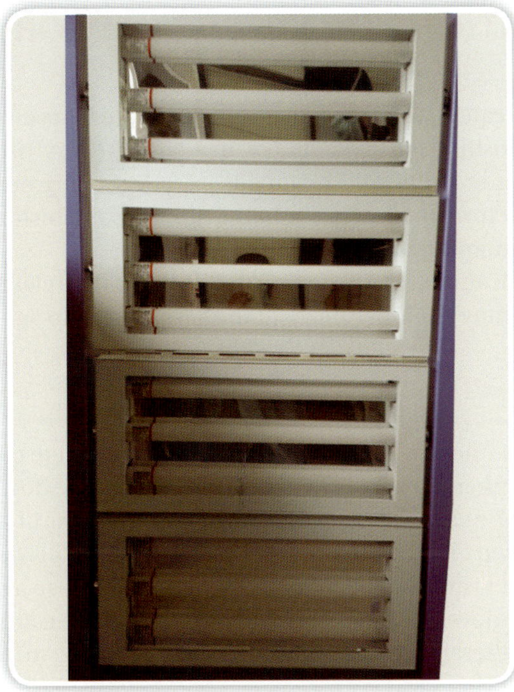

FIG. 39.3: Hand and foot NB UVB chamber

arrest. This mechanism is considered to be most important in treatment of psoriasis, with reduction in the dividing cells of basal layers as well as suprabasal epidermis.

2. UVB also induces prostaglandin release and alters cytokine expression and secretion. NBUVB decreases the expression of type 1 cytokine interferon-α and its inducers interleukin (IL)-12, IL-18 and IL-23 in the lesional skin. It has also been suggested that UVB rays reduce natural killer cell activity and also deplete the immunocompetent T-cells from the epidermis and dermis by inducing apoptosis.
3. NBUVB suppresses the functions of antigen presenting cells thus inhibiting the ability of these cells to present antigens. The newly discovered T cell subset, the Th17 cells, considered to be in the center stage of psoriasis pathogenesis are also down-regulated. Therefore, in addition to suppressive effect on keratinocytes, NBUVB also results in immunomodulation.On a per-photon basis, UVB possesses more energy than UVA but due to its shorter wavelength, it has superficial penetration and affects only epidermal keratinocytes and Langerhans cells.

INDICATIONS OF NBUVB

Phototherapy especially NBUVB acts as a bridge between topical and systemic therapies in the management of psoriasis.The indications of NBUVB in psoriasis are as follows:

1. Generalized psoriasis involving more than 10% of the body surface area.
2. Psoriasis involving limited areas of the body but not responding to topical treatment.
3. Involvement of areas that are causing physical or psychological morbidities, like hands and feet.[6]

CONTRAINDICATIONS OF NB-UVB IN PSORIASIS

These are as follows:

1. NBUVB is contraindicated in patients who have any photosensitive condition, and in those with a predisposition or are actually having a history of cutaneous malignancy. These conditions include lupus erythematosus, xeroderma pigmentosum, those who have received arsenic in any form or ionizing radiation therapy and history of previous melanoma or multiple non-melanoma skin cancers.
2. The relative contraindications may be practical difficulties like claustrophobia or inability to stand in the phototherapy chamber through the session due to age or disability.[7]

PROTOCOL

The ideal goal of any phototherapy regimen is to achieve a complete clearance of psoriasis with a minimum possible number of exposures, a low cumulative UV dose and with least possible acute as well as chronic side effects. What should be the initial dose of exposure, how frequently should a patient be exposed to phototherapy, what should be the percentage increase in the UV dose at every subsequent visit, what should be the maximum dose a patient can be subjected to and what if somebody develops adverse effects of NBUVB? The answers to these intriguing aspects of NBUVB phototherapy have largely been addressed by various studies.

INSTRUCTIONS TO THE PATIENTS

Basic instructions and education about phototherapy should be given to all patients. These include the use of eye protecting goggles, shielding genitalia in male patients and avoiding unnecessary exposure to sunlight. Protection of chronically exposed skin like face and dorsa of hands, if not involved, by using proper clothing and appropriate sunscreens should be advised. The patients should ideally be provided with pamphlets containing basic information about phototherapy.

FACTORS AFFECTING THE EFFICACY OF NBUVB

As the fluorescent UV tubes employed in phototherapy equipments are known to wear out with time, and this fact can influence the therapeutic outcome, but the most important extraneous variables that can influence the outcome of any phototherapy treatment are the spectral content of the UV source employed and UV energy incident on the patients' skin. Taylor et al. on behalf of the British Photodermatology group, have put forward some recommendations regarding calibration for optimum results of UV phototherapy. All phototherapy units should have UV radiometers to measure irradiances and the meter should be calibrated annually. Some phototherapy chambers have in-built UV radiometers and reading with this meter should match closely with the directly measured irradiance values. Measurement of irradiance every 25–50 hour of use is acceptable. However, after installation of new lamps, it should be measured after every 10–15 hour of use, as lamps when new degrade more quickly.[8]

DOSAGE

The appropriate dosage is important to increase the efficacy of NBUVB and decrease the side effects associated with NBUVB.

According to recent guidelines by the American Academy of Dermatology (AAD) for treatment of psoriasis, the initial/starting dose of NBUVB can be adjudged by skin type (not a MED-based one). In the skin type-based regimen, the initial NBUVB doses recommended are 130, 220, 260, 330, 350 and 400 mJ/cm ^{2} for skin types 1 through 6, respectively. In general,the initial dose is calculated on the basis of minimal erythema dose (MED) which should be determined prior to start of phototherapy. If MED is determined, the initial dose should be 50% of MED.

What is MED?

MED is taken as the lowest UVB dose producing defined barely perceptible erythema at the test site. MED is determined 24 hour after exposure of around 1x1cm areas on the photoprotected sites (mostly upper back/buttocks)to a pre-set test dose ladder with geometric escalation of UV dose according to skin phototype.
Note: MED-Minimal erythema dose.

In India, MED is usually not determined and a starting dose employed in few published studies seems to have underestimated the initial starting dose. There are very limited and contradictory data on MED determined on type 4/5 Indian skin.

Pai et al. has determined the average MED in type 4 skin to be 600 mJ/cm ^{2} and in type 5 skin to be 1100 mJ/cm^2. In a small series of six south Indian volunteers, Serish and Srinivas observed MED to vary widely between 150 mJ/cm ^{2} and 400 mJ/cm^2. In an another study, the average MED in Indian skin (type 4/5) was determined to be around 1,000 mJ/cm ^{2}.

The initial dose of treatment is generally 70% of the MED. Various studies have however, observed no significant difference in the near (70% of MED) vs far (35% of MED) erythemogenic doses of NBUVB as initial treatment dose in psoriasis (Hofer et al., Kleinpenning et al .). The high-dose group (70%MED) has however been found to require usually fewer treatment sessions without any significant difference in cumulative dose required to achieve final clearance.

Dose increments: In general, the dose increment in NBUVB depends on erythema response. The erythema response is assessed before the next phototherapy session and can be graded as:

Grade 1—No or mild and barely perceptible erythema
Grade 2—Moderate and well-defined asymptomatic erythema, and
Grade 3—Severe painful erythema persisting for more than 24 hour

In case there is no erythema, the dose is increased by 20% of the last dose. In the presence of grade 1 erythema, the previous dose is maintained and subsequent dose increment is reduced to 10%. In case of grade 2 erythema, postpone one treatment, repeat previous dose at next visit and reduce to 10% increment, while in case of grade 3 erythema, no treatment is offered until recovery and further treatment is given by reducing exposure dose by half and 10% increment thereafter. Studies have observed little difference in the total dose required for disease clearance in the low-increment (10%) and high-increment (20%) protocols. Moreover, the period of remission and time to relapse is also almost similar (Boztepe et al., Wainwright et al.). But both the median maximum dose and the cumulative dose required to achieve clearance/response is significantly higher with 20% escalations. The American Academy of Dermatology (AAD) recommends predetermined dose increments according to skin phototype 15, 25, 40, 45, 60 and 65 mJ/cm^2 for skin types 1 through 6, with a maximum dose of 2,000 mJ/cm for skin types 1 and 2; 3,000 mJ/cm for types 3 and 4 and 5,000 mJ/cm^2 for types 5 and 6. If pretreatment MED is determined, the dose increment should be 10% of the initial MED for the initial 20 exposures and as per physicians' discretion thereafter.[9]

The frequency of exposure to NBUVB is generally thrice to five-times a week.The efficacy of twice-weekly vs four times a week as well as three vs five times a week have been assessed in psoriasis. Twice-a-week treatment is convenient for the patient and two to three groups of patients can be treated in a week instead of one group (4/week) in a single NBUVB chamber. It has been reported that phototherapy with erythemogenic doses applied 3/week vs 5/week does not significantly change the clearance rate and duration of remission. The number of treatments and cumulative dose of UVB at clearance were significantly higher with the 5/week regimen (Dawe et al.). Similarly, Leenutaphong et al. in their comparative study of low-dose NBUVB (50% MED starting dose) with exposures 2/week vs 4/week observed that clearance rate and duration required for clearance of psoriasis were comparable in both the groups.

What to do in case of non-compliance or when a dose is missed?

If a dose is missed due to some reason or the other, NBUVB can be restarted according to the following schedule:

Less than 1 week—Maintain the last exposure dose
1-2 weeks—Restart at a dose <25% of the last dose
2-3 weeks—Restart at 50% depleted dose
More than 3 weeks interruption—Photherapy should be restarted from the previous starting dose.

How long should phototherapy be continued after achieving clearance?

In a relapsing disease like psoriasis, the duration of remission after phototherapy is important as none of the phototherapy modalities or systemic therapy is devoid of side-effects. NBUVB has gradually replaced BBUVB and is found to be equally efficacious to psoralen UVA (PUVA) in the management of psoriasis. It has been suggested that maintenance treatment with twice or once monthly exposures prolongs the duration of remission. Green et al. reported that 38% of their NBUVB-treated patients were in remission after 1 year while Collins et al. reported the corresponding figure to be 42% in their PUVA-treated patients. Post-treatment maintenance regimen (twice-weekly for the first 4 weeks and once-weekly for the next 4 weeks, totaling 12 exposures) helped 55% of the patients treated with NBUVB to remain in remission against 33% who did not receive it.[10]

SIDE EFFECTS AND COMPLICATIONS OF NB-UVB PHOTOTHERAPY

1. Erythema is a short-term acute side effect. The Incidence of erythema with NBUVB is higher than that with PUVA (varies from 10-94%). However, the incidence of therapy postponement as a result of erythema is higher with PUVA due to the persistent nature of erythema caused by it.
2. Blistering has been reported to occasionally appear at the sites of psoriatic lesions during treatment. It has been speculated that a rapid decrease in acanthosis and desquamation overpowers the protective mechanisms, namely the induction of pigmentation and increase in the thickness of stratum corneum. Appearance of plaque tenderness may be a valuable guide to impending blistering. It is recommended that the dose should be reduced to allow the nonacclimatized skin to adjust and reduce blistering.
3. Pruritus has been reported as an occasional side effect of NBUVB, although it may represent the pruritic nature of the underlying disease rather than being precipitated by NBUVB.
4. Reactivation of orolabial herpes simplex may occur and hence precautionary measures would be prudent in those who are prone to frequent relapses (role of prophylactic acyclovir?).
5. Exposure keratitis and conjunctivitis can occur following NBUVB exposure. Although cataract formation is not a problem with NBUVB as is possible with PUVA, it is better that eye protection protocol during UV exposure should be stringently followed but is not recommended.
6. Tanning: Tanning is induced by NBUVB as the duration of treatment is increased. NBUVB-induced tanning has been found to increase gradually with increasing duration of treatment, and post-treatment recovery requires at least 2–3 months.
7. Carcinogenicity: There are very scarce studies on the carcinogenic potential of NBUVB. The current available literature suggests that the cancer risk with NBUVB is probably less than that with PUVA, but is probably two to three-times more carcinogenic than BBUVB in equivalent doses. However, it is proposed that this disadvantage of NBUVB can be offset by the fact that the number of MEDs required for clearance of psoriasis is lower with NBUVB than that for BBUVB. Weischer et al. in a retrospective study involving 195 psoriasis patients receiving either BBUVB or NBUVB, suggested that neither of these modalities predispose to increased skin cancer risk. In a review of carcinogenic risk of phototherapy involving studies published in MEDLINE between 1966 and 2002, Lee et al. concluded that they could not identify any human data on the risk of non-melanoma skin cancer with NBUVB to determine the clinical relevance.[11] Thus, long-term controlled studies are needed to establish the carcinogenic potential of NBUVB.

NB-UVB VS BB-UVB IN PSORIASIS

Phototherapy or light therapy, involves exposing the skin to ultraviolet light on a regular basis and under medical supervision. Treatments are done in a doctor's office or psoriasis clinic or at home with phototherapy unit. The key to success with light therapy is consistency. UVB (a component of sunlight) is an effective treatment for psoriasis. UVB penetrates the skin and decreases/arrests the growth of affected skin cells. Treatment involves exposing the skin to an artificial UVB light source for a defined length of time on a regular schedule. This treatment is administered in a medical setting or at home.

There are two types of UVB treatments, broadband and narrowband. Narrowband UVB is, however, similar to broadband UVB in many ways,the major difference between them is that narrowband UVB light exposes patients to a very narrow range of ultraviolet light. Several studies indicate that narrowband UVB clears psoriasis faster and produces longer remissions than broadband UVB. It also may be effective with fewer treatments per week than broadband UVB.

During UVB treatment,the psoriasis may worsen temporarily (erythema and itching are the most common side effects) and occasional flares may occur before improving. These reactions, however, tend to resolve with continued treatment.

To avoid further irritation, the amount of UVB administered should be reduced.

UVB has been combined with various topical and/or systemic antipsoriatic agents to enhance efficacy, but some of these may increase photosensitivity and burning, or shorten remission.The combination, however, has the advantage of less incidence of side effects due to lower cumulative doses of either agent when used in combination.[12,13]

Fluorescent lamps emitting light in the BBUVB range have broad spectral emission with some proportion (about 5.5%) of wavelength within the UVC range (<290 nm). In addition to these conventional BBUVB lamps, fluorescent lamps with little emission in the UVC range (0.5%) are also available, the so-called selective broadband UVB (UV6). NBUVB lamps emit 0.1% radiations below 290 nm.

Majority of the studies comparing the efficacy of BBUVB and NBUVB in psoriasis have demonstrated that NBUVB is better than BBUVB, with maximal clearance response being produced after fewer treatments. Studies have also demonstrated that satisfactory response and total duration of therapy are shorter with NBUVB. The conclusion of a recent meta-analysis of controlled studies was also similar. The main limitations with NBUVB is longer exposure time per session and four to six-times higher doses required to generate an equi-erythemogenic effect.[14]

There are only few studies comparing selective ultraviolet B (SUV, little emission below 290 nm) with NBUVB. In one side-to-side comparison study of NBUVB with SUV in combination with the Ingram regimen, the results were comparable in 60% of the patients, and in the rest, NBUVB was found to be more effective. In an another side-to-side comparison study of NBUVB and SUV, both the modalities were compared in 23 patients. In 13 patients, dithranol was applied on both the treatment sides, in addition according to the modified Ingram regimen. In 20 patients, NBUVB was found to be significantly more efficacious. The exposure times were comparable between the groups. In a recent randomized comparative study, both the modalities were found to be comparable, with 56% in the NBUVB group and 40% in the SUV group achieving clearance, with a median number of exposures of 28.4 for NBUVB and 30.4 for SUV.[15] Thus, NBUVB is clearly more effective than selective ultraviolet B (SUV).

NB-UVB VS PUVA IN PSORIASIS

Various studies have compared the efficacy of NBUVB and PUVA in the management of psoriasis.

Van Weelden et al.[16] in their side-to-side comparative study, observed no significant difference between the overall therapeutic effectiveness of NBUVB and PUVA in the clearance of psoriatic plaques. The study was performed on 10 patients. In three cases, PUVA was more effective than NBUVB, in two cases NBUVB was better than PUVA and in the remaining five cases, there was no difference.

In an open, nonrandomized, intraindividually controlled paired comparison study in 25 patients, NBUVB was found to be as effective as PUVA, but PUVA gave better results in patients with high PASI scores.The overall reduction in PASI was 84% in the NBUVB group and 89% in the PUVA group.

Markham et al. performed a randomized controlled study in 54 patients, with 29 patients receiving NBUVB (three-times a week) and 25 being administered oral PUVA (twice weekly). Those in the PUVA group required significantly fewer treatments for clearance. However, there was no statistically significant difference in the number of days to clearance or period of remission.

Gordon et al.[17] in their study involving 100 patients (with 51 receiving NBUVB and 41 PUVA), observed significantly better results with PUVA than NBUVB. In the PUVA group, 84% had clearance of lesions with a mean of 16.7 exposures while in the NBUVB group 63% had clearance of lesions with a mean of 25.3 exposures. Moreover, the remission rate was three-times at 6 months for PUVA than for NBUVB. In this study, only 12% of those treated with NBUVB were clear of Psoriasis 6 months after treatment compared with 35% of those treated with PUVA. Other studies, have also documented a longer remission period with PUVA as compared to NBUVB, which is one of the greatest disadvantages of NBUVB.

Yones et al. performed a double-blind placebo controlled study on 93 patients, with 47 receiving NBUVB and 46 PUVA. In the PUVA group, 84% patients achieved clearance after 17 exposures while in the NBUVB group 65% patients achieved clearance after a mean of 28.5 exposures. At 6 months post-treatment, 68% and 35% patients in the corresponding groups were in remission. In a study from India, Kaur et al.[18] found complete clearance of the lesions in 75% of the patients in the PUVA group ($n = 16$) and 64% in the NBUVB group ($n = 17$).

Thus, all the studies are of the opinion that both the modalities (NBUVB and PUVA) induce comparable clearance in psoriasis. However, the duration of remission may be longer with PUVA as concluded by various studies.

Certain advantages of NBUVB which score over PUVA are no or minimal risk of carcinogenesis compared with PUVA, safety of its use in children and pregnant patients, absence of drug-related (psoralen intake) side effects and no requirement of post-treatment eye protection.

COMBINATION REGIMENS WITH NB-UVB

NBUVB has been used in combination with topical and systemic antipsoriatic agents as well as biological agents. Combination therapy has practical benefits viz, rapid response to treatment and lower incidence of side effects since the cumulative dose of either drug is reduced when used in combination.

1. *NBUVB with topical steroids:* The role of topical corticosteroids in conjunction with UVB has been controversial. Earlier reports suggested a fast clearance of disease in patients treated with this combination. A subsequent study has suggested an increased relapse rate. Efficacy of topical dithranol in combination with NBUVB has been assessed by Carrozza et al., and it was observed that the combination resulted in a significant decrease in disease severity. The cumulative UV dose was similar or lower to that found for NBUVB alone.[19]
2. *NBUVB with Vitamin D3 analogues:* The available current literature suggests the possible synergistic effect of the combination of NBUVB and vitamin D3 analogues in the clearance of psoriasis, but studies have yielded variable results. Calcipotriol has been suggested to have UVB-sparing effects when used in combination in the treatment of psoriasis. It is a well-known fact that light exposure can degrade vitamin D3 analogues and thus when used in combination, application of vitamin D3 analogues should follow phototherapy. However, Adachi et al. is of the contrary opinion that no such deleterious effect of PUVA or NBUVB on vitamin D3 analogues are seen. Messer et al. in their study suggested that NBUVB in combination with pretreatment tacalcitol is superior to either monotherapy alone. The combination regimen in their study led to >50% reduction in PASI in 86% of the lesions while in a side-to-side comparison study tacalcitol monotherapy led to a similar improvement in 38% of the lesions. In contrast, Brands et al. observed that addition of calcipotriol to low-dose NBUVB does not have any added therapeutic benefit, but Rim et al. observed more rapid clearance of psoriasis with combination regimen at the early stage while the final and total cumulative dose of NBUVB in the combination group was slightly lower, although not statistically significant. The combination of NBUVB with either calcitriol or dithranol has been found to be equally effective. However, patients usually prefer calcitriol over dithranol, when allowed to choose between the two due to staining properties and other side effects of dithranol.[20]
3. *NBUVB with Psoralens:* Both topical and systemic psoralens, have been found to enhance the efficacy of NBUVB in clearing psoriatic plaques. In a side-to-side comparison of NBUVB vs combination of NBUVB and psoralens (PUVB) involving 10 patients, lesions cleared earlier in the PUVB-treated side in eight of the nine patients (89%) who completed the study. In a subsequent study of the comparison of PUVB and PUVA from the same center which involved 100 patients, it was concluded that PUVB is slightly more effective than PUVA. The median number of exposures for clearance was 16.5 for PUVA and 15 for PUVB.The incidence of erythema was comparable in both the groups. Topical 8-methoxypsoralen has been demonstrated to augment the efficacy of NBUVB (Seckin et al.). The combination has been suggested to lead to greater and earlier improvement than NBUVB alone. The overall clearance rate is also noted to be higher with the combination, however, side effects are more common with the combination and pigmentation is the most common adverse effect.[21]
4. *NBUVB with cytotoxic agents (methotrexate and cyclosporine):* Various short-term studies have shown the augmented efficacy of the combination of NBUVB and methotrexate/cyclosporine. In a study, a combination of methotrexate 15 mg/week and NBUVB was found to be more effective than NBUVB alone. In a randomized, placebo-controlled study by Asawanonda et al., methotrexate (15 mg/week) or placebo was given for 3 weeks before standard NBUVB was started. It was observed that the median time for clearance in the combination group was 4 weeks, which was significantly shorter than that in the NBUVB monotherapy group. Similarly, a comparative study of sequential cyclosporine and NBUVB vs NBUVB treatment

alone indicated that the former (cyclosporine with NBUVB) is better in the management of psoriasis.The main advantages of the combination were less NBUVB dosage and exposure and decreased dose of cyclosporine and rapid clearance of the psoriatic plaques and subjective symptoms.The major disadvantage of the combination of NBUVB with cytotoxic agents is the heightened risk of skin cancers, thus long-term studies are needed. [22]

5. *NBUVB with acitretin:* Various studies have demonstrated that the combination of acitretin and NBUVB is having a synergistic effect in the management of psoriasis. In one study, forty patients who failed to respond to BBUVB, NBUVB, acitretin monotherapy or a combination of BBUVB and acitretin, were treated with a combination of acitretin (25 mg/day) and NBUVB. More than 75% improvement from baseline was noticed in 72.5% patients while only 12.5% patients had less than 50% improvement.The main advantage of this combination is that the reduced doses of each therapy minimizes the acute and chronic side effects associated with each therapy (acitretin can mitigate the carcinogenic potential of NBUVB).[23]
6. *NBUVB with biological agents:* The available current literature suggests that efalizumab is effective in only 1/3rd of the patients. Addition of NBUVB to efalizumab in the first 4 weeks of the 6-months treatment schedule of efalizumab (1 mg/kg/week) in one study has been shown to result in clearance of psoriatic plaques in approximately 70% of the patients. In another study, the combination of NBUVB thrice a week and efalizumab 1 mg/kg/week achieved PASI 75 in 65% of the patients after 12 weeks of treatment.The combination of NBUVB and etanercept is also found to have a synergistic effect. In a study where NBUVB thrice-a-week was combined with etanercept 50 mg twice-a-week, PASI 75 was achieved in 84.9% of the patients and PASI 100 was achieved in 26% of the patients. Scheinfeld has reported two treatment-resistant cases of psoriasis who did not respond to methotrexate and UVB alone but responded to the combination of alefacept followed by NBUVB leading to complete clearance of disease, thus documenting the synergistic effects of the combination.[24]

PRETREATMENT EMOLLIENT APPLICATION

Various studies on pretreatment application of emollients before broadband UVB has shown that it can rapidly clear psoriasis due to synergistic effects. Thus similar studies were then undertaken in case of NBUVB also. It is a proven fact that for phototherapy to produce maximal effects in psoriasis, it should penetrate sufficiently into the skin, since in psoriasis, the scales form multiple air-corneocyte interfaces that increase reflectance of the optic radiations. Thus, the application of a suitable emollient before light exposure can effectively reduce these air-corneocyte interfaces, thus enhancing the transmission of UV radiation through the epidermis. One of the major advantages of pretreatment application of emollients is that the acute (erythema, blistering) and chronic side effects (skin cancers) of phototherapy are reduced to a great extent. However, the most suitable emollients are those that are non-photosensitizing and non-UV absorbing, and the monochromatic protection factor of such emollients should be <1.2 to avoid a reduction in UV transmission.Examples of such emollients are vaseline, glycerine, mineral oil, 5% oleic acid, etc. However, every emollient is not suitable for pretreatment application, i.e. salicylic acid-containing agents like dithranol, coal tar, etc., as they impart a photoprotective effect, thus decreasing the efficacy of phototherapy.[25]

RECENT DEVELOPMENTS

One of the major disadvantages of conventional phototherapy in whole-body chambers or phototherapy panels is the unnecessary exposure of the unaffected normal skin to ultraviolet light. This also prevents the use of higher doses of phototherapy, particularly in resistant lesions of psoriasis, so as to achieve rapid clearance of disease. The other drawbacks of the conventional phototherapy chambers are lengthy individual treatment sessions, frequent clinic visits, large space required to accommodate the bulky machines and intimidation of young patients with heavy size and closed chambers. In order to circumvent these side effects of conventional phototherapy, the focuss has been shifted to targeted phototherapy, which is used to treat particularly the localized disease (<10% body surface area). Since the output is higher from these devices, thus higher dose can be delivered in a shorter time resulting in rapid clearance of the psoriatic plaques. Intense pulsed light, excimer laser, photodynamic therapy and UV light-based source are some of the forms of targeted phototherapy which are used in psoriasis and other varied indications.The source of UV light in these targeted phototherapy devices is similar to the conventional devices, however, the light is delivered directly onto the lesions by fiber optic cables, and it has been suggested that more number of lesions get cleared with increasing the fluence of UVB (Asawanonda et al.). Asymptomatic erythema and hyperpigmentation are the most common side effects. It is believed that NBUVB may not be an appropriate option for palmoplantar lesions or nail psoriasis since the penetration of NBUVB is rather superficial, but Campolmi et al. has observed that palmoplantar lesions respond better and the time to relapse is longer for palmoplantar lesions compared with other areas.[26]

CONCLUSION

NBUVB has been found to be a relatively safer but comparatively effective alternative to PUVA in in the management of psoriasis since its introduction about two decades back. NBUVB has the advantage that it can be used in combination with both topical and systemic immunosuppressive agents in the management of psoriasis. Targeted NBUVB in combination with topical 0.1% 8-methoxypsoralen cream has been found to be much more efficacious in clearing psoriatic lesions compared with targeted phototherapy alone. The exact dosimetry of NBUVB is yet to be determined; the most commonly employed dosing regimen is 70% MED as starting dose with 20% dose increments till minimal perceptible erythema is elicited. The recent development of targeted phototherapy has the prospect of clearing even resistant psoriatic lesions and lesions at inaccessible sites in a shorter period of time.[27]

Points to Remember

- Targeted phototherapy has been developed to treat localized disease (<10% body surface area) keeping the drawbacks of conventional phototherapy in mind
- NBUVB has been found to be a comparatively effective and relatively safer alternative to PUVA in more than two decades of use in the management of psoriasis
- Targeted NBUVB (dose applied at four-times MED) in combination with topical 0.1% 8-methoxypsoralen cream has been found to be much more efficacious in clearing psoriatic lesions compared with targeted phototherapy alone

Note: NBUVB—Narrowband ultraviolet B; PUVA—Psoralen with Ultravoilet A; MED—Minimal erythema dose; PUVB—Narrowband UVB with psoralens

REFERENCES

1. Dogra S, Kanwar AJ. Narrowband UVB phototherapy in dermatology. Indian J Dermatol Venereol Leprol. 2004;70:205-9.
2. Wiskemann A. UVB- phototherapie der psoriasis mit einer fur die PUVA- therapie entwickelten stehbox. Z Hautzkr. 1978;53:633-6.
3. Parrish JA, Jaenicke KF. Action spectrum for phototherapy of psoriasis. J Invest Dermatol. 1981;76:359-62.
4. van Weelden H, De La Faille HB, Young E, van der Leun JC. A new development in UVB phototherapy for psoriasis. Br J Dermatol. 1988;119:11-9.
5. Green C, Ferguson J, Lakshmipathi T, Johnson BE. 311 nm UVB phtotherapy- an effective treatment for psoriasis. Br J Dermatol. 1988;119:691-96.
6. Honigsmann H, Ortel B. Phototherapy and photochemotherapy. In: Photodermatology. Hawk JL, editor. Arnold London; 1999. p. 223-40.
7. Lever LR, Farr PM. Skin cancers or premalignant lesions occur in half of high dose PUVA patients. Br J Dermatol 1994;131:215-9.
8. Parrish JA, Jaenicke KF. Action spectrum of phototherapy of psoriasis. J Invest Dermatol. 1981;76:359-62.
9. Boztepe G, Akinci H, Sahin S, Karaduman A, Ersoy Evans S, Erkin G, *et al.* In search of an optimal dose escalation for narrowband UVB phototherapy: Is it time to quit 20% dose increments? J Am Acad Dermatol. 2006;55:269-71.
10. Srinivas CR, Shenoi SD, Pai S. Psoralens. Indian J Dermatol Venereol Leprol. 1997;63:276-87.
11. Marco Petrazzuoli. Advances in phototherapy. Curr Probl Dermatol. Nov/Dec. 2000;282-6.
12. Goekerman WH. The treatment of psoriasis. Northwest Med. 1925;24:229-31.
13. An appraisal of narrowband (TL-01) UVB phototherapy. British Photoderamtology Group Workshop report. Br J Dermatol. 1997;137:327-30.
14. British Photodermatology Group: An appraisal of narrowband UVB phototherapy: British Photodermatology Group Workshop Report (April, 1996). Br J Dermatol. 1997;137:327-30.
15. Honigsmann H, Szeimies RM, Knobler R, et al. Photochemotherapy and Photodynamic Therapy, In: Dermatology in General Medicine, 5th edn, Edited by Fitzpatrick et al. McGraw Hill Book Company: New York; 1999.2880-2900.
16. Van Welden H, Baart de la Faille H, Young E, van der Leun JC. Comparison of narrowband UV-B phototherapy and PUVA photochemotherapy in the treatment of psoriasis. Acta Derm Venereol. 1990;70:212-5.
17. Gordon PM, Diffey BL, Matthews JN, Farr PM. A randomized comparison of narrowband TL-01 phototherapy and PUVA photochemotherapy for psoriasis. J Arn Acad Dermatol. 1999;41:728-32.
18. Kaur J, Shrama VK, Sethuraman G, Tejasvi T. Comparison of the efficacy of psoralen ultraviolet A with narrowband ultraviolet B phototherapy for the treatment of chronic plaque psoriasis in patients with skin types 4 and 5. Clin Exp Dermatol. 2008;33:513-5.
19. Dover JS, McEvoy MT, Rosen CF, Arndt KA, Stern RS. Are topical corticosteroids useful in phototherapy for psoriasis? J Am Acad Dermatol. 1989;20:748-54.
20. Woo WK, McKenna KE. Combination TL01 ultraviolet B phototherapy and topical calcipotriol for psoriasis: A prospective randomized placebo-controlled clinical trial. Br J Dermatol. 2003;149:146-50.
21. Sakuntabhai A, Diffey BL, Farr PM. Response of psoriasis to psoralen- UVB photochemotherapy. Br J Dermatol. 1993;128:296-300.
22. Asawanonda P, Nateetongrungsak Y. Methotrexate plus narrowband UVB phototherapy versus narrowband UVB phototherapy alone in the treatment of plaque-type psoriasis: a randomized, placebo-controlled study. J Am Acad Dermatol. 2006;54:1013-8.
23. Spuls PI, Rozenblit M, Lebwohl M. Retrospective study of the efficacy of narrowband UVB and acitretin. J Dermatolog Treat. 2003;14:17-20.

24. Zane C, Capezzera R, Venturini M, Sala R, Facchinetti E, Pedretti A, *et al.* A short cycle of narrowband UVB phototherapy in the early phase of long-term efalizumab can provide a quicker remission of moderate and severe psoriasis: A pilot study. Dermatology. 2009;218:321-6.
25. Penven K, Leroy D, Verneuil L, Faguer K, Dompmartin A. Evaluation of Vaseline oil applied prior to UVB TL01 phototherapy in the treatment of psoriasis. Photodermatol Photoimmunol Photomed. 2005;21:138-41.
26. Mysore V. Targeted phototherapy. Indian J Dermatol Venereol Leprol. 2009;75:119-27.
27. Lotti T, Rossi R, Campolmi P. Targeted UV-B phototherapy: When and why to start. Arch Dermatol. 2006;142:933-34.

Chapter

40

Targeted Phototherapy in Psoriasis

Phototherapy deals with the use of nonionizing electromagnetic radiation to bring about a beneficial effect on a particular disease. Phototherapy is used for a wide variety of skin diseases. PUVA or Psoralens with UV-A light exposure is an established therapy for psoriasis, but there is a well-documenated risk of melanoma and non-melanoma skin cancer. Narrowband ultraviolet-B (NBUVB) therapy has a lower carcinogenic risk, has equal therapeutic potential and is considerably safe in the long-term than PUVA. There has been a considerable progress in cellular and cutaneous photobiology leading to improved understanding of different photodermatoses and their treatment.

The last two decades have seen significant technological advances in light therapy of psoriasis, expanding the options while treating a patient who needs phototherapy. The most important of these advances have been narrowband ultraviolet B (NBUVB-311 nm) phototherapy and, more recently, targeted phototherapy.[1]

WHY DO WE NEED TARGETED PHOTOTHERAPY?[2,3]

The reasons why we need targeted phototherapy are summarized further in this chapter. (Disadvantages of conventional phototherapy and advantages of targeted phototherapy).

Disadvantages of Conventional Phototherapy

Conventional phototherapy consists of the use of light energy delivered by tube lights to the affected area. Different machines used for this purpose include whole body cabinets, hand and foot machines, scalp machines, etc.These machines have the following disadvantages:

1. Exposure of uninvolved areas.
2. Slow delivery system and lengthy treatment sessions.
3. Multiple and frequent visits to the hospital/clinic.
4. Difficulty in treating certain areas, such as genitalia, oral mucosa, ears, etc.
5. Difficulty in treating children who may feel intimidated by the large machines.
6. Large office space required to keep the bulky machines.

A new technique called targeted phototherapy which seeks to overcome these disadvantages has now become available. Also called concentrated phototherapy, focused phototherapy, microphototherapy, this modality involves delivery of light energy directly focused on, or targeted at, the lesion through special delivery mechanisms, such as fiber-optic cables. The term 'targeted phototherapy' includes different technologies, such as excimer laser, intense pulse light systems, and UV light sources with improved hand-held delivery systems.

Advantages of Targeted Phototherapy

The various advantages of targeted phototherapy are discussed below:

a. Since the affected sites are only exposed and unexposed areas are spared, thus the acute side effects, such as erythema and long-term risk of skin cancer over unaffected skin are minimized.
b. Shortened duration of treatment because of the quick delivery of energy at the affected sites only.
c. Higher doses of energy can be delivered selectively to the lesions, thereby enhancing efficacy and achieving faster response.
d. Targeted phototherapy has been claimed to shorten the duration of treatment, leading to less frequent visits to clinic, and hence increasing the productive time and decreasing the inconvenience for the patient.
e. Difficult areas, such as scalp, nose, genitals, oral mucosa and ears can be treated due to maneuverability of the hand piece.
f. Ease of administration for children as the delivery is hand-held.
g. Targeted phototherapy machines occupy less space.

Disadvantages of Targeted Phototherapy

Targeted phototherapy devices have certain disadvantages, viz, that are discussed below:

a. Targeted phototherapy machines are more expensive.
b. Targeted phototherapy is not adequate to treat extensive areas in view of the cost of treatment and time involved in treatment.
c. Targeted phototherapy is not recommended for use if lesions occur over more than 10% of the body surface area.

MECHANISM OF ACTION

Ultravoilet light (UV light) has been shown to have several effects on both epidermal and dermal cells, which explains its efficacy in treatment of cutaneous diseases, such as psoriasis, vitiligo, and lymphoma. Apoptotic mechanisms may be involved in the destruction of susceptible epidermal and dermal cells by UV light. UVB radiation has been shown to induce DNA damage and pyrimidine dimer formation, result in induction of alteration in cytokine production, local immunosuppression, stimulation of melanocyte-stimulating hormone, increased melanocyte proliferation, and melanogenesis. UVB radiation also enhances production of vitamin D metabolites, which stimulate melanogenesis. UVA radiation may also produce similar effects. Most targeted phototherapy devices (laser or nonlaser type) emit radiation in the UVB range, with peak emission in the narrowband wavelength (around 308-311 nm), while some light-based nonlaser machines emit UVA radiation also. Hence mechanisms of action of targeted phototherapy systems are similar to those in conventional UVB/UVA therapy. Targeted phototherapy may induce all these effects mentioned above in a more aggressive way, because of the delivery of super erythemogenic doses of radiation. It has also been suggested that their enhanced efficacy may be due to their ability to deliver the energy to deeper dermal levels, and targeted therapy may therefore affect hidden target cells, such as melanocytes.[4,5]

DIFFERENT TYPES OF TARGETED PHOTOTHERAPIES

Targeted phototherapy may be achieved by different sources, such as excimer laser, IPL (excimer light), and UV light.

Excimer Laser[6]

An excimer laser (or exciplex laser) is a form of ultraviolet laser which is commonly used in the production of microelectronic devices, eye surgery, and micromachining. The term excimer is short for 'excited dimer', while exciplex is short form for 'excited complex'. Most excimer lasers are of the noble gas halide type, for which the term excimer is strictly speaking a misnomer (since a dimer refers to a molecule of two identical or similar parts); hence the correct name which is less commonly used for such lasers is exciplex laser.

Excimer laser was first used in medicine for its ability to produce cold tissue ablation, but later found applications in cardiology, ophthalmology, orthopedics, and dermatology. The word 'excimer' refers to 'excited dimer.' These lasers operate in the ultraviolet range, and examples include the 193-nm argon-fluoride; 248-nm krypton-fluoride; 351-nm xenon-fluoride; and of particular interest to dermatology, the 308-nm xenon-chloride laser. These lasers utilize a mixture of a noble gas and a halogen as a lasing material. The pulse repetition rate of the laser can be set up to 200 Hz with 3mJ/cm^2 of energy per pulse. A pilot study in 2002 showed significant benefits in vitiligo. Twenty-nine patches of vitiligo from 18 patients were treated 3 times a week for a maximum of 12 times with excimer laser, with parameters 120-nanosecond, 20-Hz pulse with a 10×10-mm spot size and a power output of 60 mW of laser light. Exposure time was 2 seconds, increased by 2 seconds at every other visit. Twenty three vitiligo patches had 6 treatments, with some repigmentation in 57% of the treated patches. Eleven vitiligo patches from 6 patients had 12 treatments, with some repigmentation in 82% of the treated patches. Lesions which were previously resistant to treatment with other modalities also responded to excimer laser. The study concluded that the degree of repigmentation in a period of 2 to 4 weeks is much higher than that achieved with any other present vitiligo therapy. The xenon-chloride excimer laser may represent a new treatment modality for the management of stable vitiligo. These results were confirmed by other studies, which showed benefit with excimer laser in patients of localized vitiligo who had been unsuccessfully treated with other modalities of treatment.

In psoriasis, the efficacy of excimer laser has been confirmed by several reports. Localized resistant lesions of psoriasis over elbows and knees have been reported to clear with 1-3 exposures, with moderately long periods of remission. Scalp psoriasis has been shown to respond as well. In a survey which studied patient satisfaction, 55% of patients reported overall satisfaction and 25% reported that laser treatments were better than any other treatment they had tried. Side effects reported, though usually mild, included burning pain during and after treatment, severe erythema, and blistering of the skin. The blistering response may raise a problem for patients. Controlled trials are however, needed.

Excimer laser machines, however, have several disadvantages, such as high-cost, huge weight and bulk, and difficulties in maintenance. Despite its introduction in 2002, the technology is available only in a few centers at present.

Monochromatic Excimer Light(IPL) Therapy[7]

Phototherapy is a mainstay of vitiligo treatment and has varying rates of efficacy. Narrowband ultraviolet B (NB-UVB) and UVA have been used for decades, but it is only recently that monochromatic excimer light (MEL) has been developed for use in dermatology and tried in the treatment of vitiligo. The specific 308-nm radiation wavelength is delivered in a targeted form by the xenon-chloride excimer laser and is also available in an incoherent form that is commonly referred to as the excimer lamp. MEL administered by both laser and lamp has shown efficacy superior to NB-UVB for the treatment of vitiligo and has been demonstrated to induce more changes at the cellular level than conventional UVB modalities. Other forms of targeted light therapy have been introduced, such as IPL therapy with wavelength of 304 nm (excilite: Deka) and 308 nm (Pxlite). These machines are less bulky, cheaper, and have a comparatively larger treatment surface in contrast to excimer laser. Several studies have been published which demonstrate their efficacy.[5]

Light-Based (Nonlaser, Non-IPL) Targeted Phototherapy[8]

Sallman, Theralight, multilight, curelight, Bioskin and B-clear phototherapy are some of the advances in technology which have now permitted delivery of conventional noncoherent light (broadband or narrowband light) selectively to the target lesions. Most of these machines use a conventional high-pressure burner emitting UV light and fiber-optic cable systems to deliver energy directly to the affected sites.Their spot sizes range from 1 to 3 cm.These machines have multiple delivery programs and automatic calibration for quick delivery of predetermined dosages, so that the treatment time is short.They are considerably smaller in size than the laser machines, with less maintenance problems, and are also cheaper. An added advantage of some of these machines over the excimer light or laser is that both UVA and UVB therapeutic ranges are available. Several studies have been published on the efficacy of these systems in psoriasis and vitiligo.

Dualight

Dualight provides both UVA and UVB therapeutic ranges within one system for increased versatility. It has an easy to use system interface for UVA and UVB settings as well as minimal erythema dose (MED) and minimal phototoxic dose (MPD) automatic phototest mode. It has a built-in calibrating port for easy automated calibration. Previously called Theralight, it emits both UVA radiation in the range 330–380 nm and UVB in the range 290–330 nm with peak at 303 nm. The system has a 2-meter long fiber-optic delivery system, with a spot size of 4 cm^2. UVA intensity is 10–550 mW/cm^2 for 3.63-cm^2 exit aperture, while UVB intensity is 50–250 mW/cm^2 for 3.63 cm^2 exit aperture. Its patented square aperture handpiece design provides an unobstructed view. It is light weight to reduce operator fatigue, and has a flexible light liquid guide for easy access to areas difficult to reach.

B Clear Targeted Photoclearing System

The B clear targeted photoclearing system, is an ultraviolet light source and energy delivery system that provides targeted energy to the treatment site while avoiding unnecessary exposure of the nonaffected sites.The light source is contained within a protective console. The complete system also includes a handpiece connected to the console via an umbilical.The timing and dosing parameters and an interface to other system features are controlled from a display panel on the console. The delivery system allows UVB light to pass through the handpiece to selectively target skin and nail lesions without exposure to the healthy skin.

B clear system is a mercury-based noncoherent UVB radiation with therapeutic wavelength of 290–320 nm and pulse width of 0.5–2.0 seconds. Fluence ranges from 50 to 800 mJ/cm^2 in increments of 10 mJ/cm^2. Its disadvantage is that only UVB range is available, unlike Dualight, which delivers both UVA and UVB therapeutic ranges.[9]

Bioskin or Latest Cold-Light Generation Microphototherapy

It is a new sophisticated light emitting equipment of UVB rays (311nm) which has been tried in the treatment of vitiligo. It is probably the latest generation microphototherapy, performed with an innovative equipment which emits UVB in a specific and selective way to stimulate dormant melanocytes. Lotti et al. has reported efficacy of a targeted narrowband UVB device in vitiligo in 1999. Bioskin consists of a mercury arc lamp with wavelength 280–320 nm and peak at 311 nm and a delivery system consisting of liquid-component optical fiber with spot size 1 cm in diameter. In one study, 75% repigmentation was achieved in 5 of the 8 patients with segmental vitiligo, after 6 months treatment. Another study done on large scale in 734 patients showed 75% or more improvement in nearly 70% of the patients and total repigmentation in 21% of the subjects. No patient showed acute or chronic side effects.[10]

CONCLUSION

The role of targeted phototherapy in diseases, such as vitiligo, psoriasis, acne and in new indications, such as stretch marks is continuing to evolve. A new low-level helium neon laser system has been reported to be effective in segmental vitiligo. It is obvious that both targeted laser and nonlaser phototherapies represent exciting advances in dermatology.[11]

Points to Remember

- Most targeted phototherapy devices (laser or nonlaser type) emit radiation in the UVB range, with peak emission in the narrowband wavelength (around 308-311 nm)
- Targeted phototherapy may be achieved by different sources, such as excimer laser, IPL (excimer light), and UV light
- The role of this modality both in diseases, such as vitiligo, psoriasis and also in new indications, such as acne and stretch marks continues to evolve
- Targeted phototherapy is devoid of the side effects of conventional phototherapy

Note: UV light—Ultravoilet light; MEL—Monochromatic excimer light

REFERENCES

1. Venkataram Mysore.Targeted phototherapy in psoriasis. IJDVL. 2009;75 (2):119-125.
2. Diffey BL. Ultraviolet phototherapy of skin diseases. Physics and Engineering in Medicine in the New Millennium, IPEM; 2000. p. 65-7.
3. Bethea D, Fullmer B, Syed S, Seltzer G, Tiano J, Rischko C, et al. Psoralen photobiology and photochemotherapy: 50 years of science and medicine. J Dermatol Sci. 1999;19:78-88.
4. Grimes PE. Advances in the treatment of vitiligo: Targeted phototherapy. Cosm Dermatol. 2003;16:18-22 .
5. De Gruijl FR. Long-term side effects and carcinogenesis risk in UVB therapy. In Hongismann H, Jori G, Young AR, editors. The Fundamental Basis of Phototherapy, OEMF spa, Italy 1996. p. 153-70.
6. Kaur M, Oliver B, Hu J, Feldman SR. Nonlaser UVB-targeted phototherapy treatment of psoriasis. Cutis. 2006;78:200-3.
7. Asawanonda P, Anderson RR, Chang Y, Taylor CR. 308-nm excimer laser for the treatment of psoriasis: A dose-response study Arch Dermatol. 2000;136:619-24.
8. Aubin F, Vigan M, Puzenat E, Blanc D, Drobacheff C, Deprez P, et al. Evaluation of a novel 308-nm monochromatic excimer light delivery system in dermatology: A pilot study in different chronic localized dermatoses. Br J Dermatol. 2005;152:99-103.
9. Hamzavi I, Lui H. Using light in dermatology: An update on lasers, ultraviolet phototherapy, and photodynamic therapy. Dermatol Clin. 2005;23:199-207.
10. Gilles PR. Technical evaluation of fibre optically delivered light for lesion targeted high dosage UVB phototherapy B-clear application note 2 Lumenis inhouse publication 2002.
11. Lotti TM, Menchini G, Andreassi L. UV-B radiation microphototherapy: An elective treatment for segmental vitiligo. J Eur Acad Dermatol Venereol. 1999;13:102-8.

Chapter

41 Biological Agents for Psoriasis

Psoriasis is a common chronic immune-mediated skin disease characterized by cutaneous inflammation and epidermal hyperproliferation. Lesions can appear on any part of the skin, but are particularly seen in the region of scalp, sacral area, and over the extensor aspect of knees and elbows.

Systemic psoralens in conjunction with ultraviolet light (PUVA) is the phototherapy treatment of first choice for extensive psoriasis. PUVA is a form of photochemotherapy that combines the use of a psoralen (e.g. methoxsalen) with ultraviolet A light in the range of 320–400 nm. PUVA is highly effective in the treatment of psoriasis with resolution of skin lesions in over 85 % of patients after 20–30 treatments. Ultravoilet-B (UVB) phototherapy may be given alone or in combination with tar or dithranol.[1]

Other systemic treatments for psoriasis include methotrexate, retinoids and cyclosporine. But these treatment modalities are contraindicated in pregnancy and require close monitoring.[2]

Biologics or biological agents are protein molecules which are used in various diseases to target the specific points in the immunopathogenesis of diseases. These molecules are produced by recombinant DNA technology. Since these molecules bind to the specific targets without interfering with rest of the pathogenetic pathways, hence the side-effects seen with these agents are also less. On the contrary, the various immunosuppressive agents (e.g. methotrexate, cyclosporine, etc.) used in the treatment of psoriasis, although are characterized by a broader spectrum of action, are equally more toxic with greater range of side effects.[3]

CLASSIFICATION

Biologics are divided into three groups:

1. Recombinant human cytokines and growth factors.
2. Monoclonal antibodies.
3. Fusion antibody proteins.

Recombinant Human Cytokines and Growth Factors

These include interferon α (IFNα), interferon γ (IFNγ), interleukin 1 receptor antagonist (IL1Ra), interleukin 2 (IL-2), interleukin 4 (rhIL-4), interleukin 10 (rhIL-10), interleukin 11 (rhIL-11), granulocyte macrophage colony stimulating factor (GM-CSF) and platelet-derived growth factor (PDGF).

Monoclonal Antibodies

The principal monoclonal antibodies with therapeutic relevance in psoriasis are:

- Anti-TNFα: Infliximab, Adalimumab, Certolizumab and Golimumab
- Anti-LFA1: Efalizumab
- Anti-CD20: Rituximab
- Anti-IL-12 and anti-IL-23 monoclonal antibody: Ustekinumab
- Anti-CD2 antibody: Siplizumab
- Anti-CD4 antibody: Orthoclone (OKTcdr4a)
- Anti-CD25 antibodies: Basiliximab, Daclizumab
- Anti-CD80r: Galiximab (IDEC 114)
- Anti-IgE: Omalizumab.

Fusion Antibody Proteins

The fusion antibody proteins which have been studied extensively in psoriasis are: etanercept, alefacept, abatacept and denileukin diftitox.

Guidelines on psoriasis from the Finnish Medical Society[4] (2005) state that biologicals such as alefacept, efalizumab, etanercept and infliximab may have a role in the treament of moderate to severe psoriasis refractory to other systemic treatments or when other systemic treatments are contraindicated or unsuitable.

Guidelines on psoriasis from the British Association of Dermatologists (BAD guidelines, 2005) state that, at present, the risks and benefits of antitumor necrosis factor (anti-TNF) agents, or efalizumab, relative to standard systemic therapy are unknown. The guidelines state that early and widespread use of these agents in uncomplicated moderate to severe psoriasis is inappropriate and is not supported by the recommended indications for etanercept or efalizumab.

The British Association of Dermatologists guidelines (BAD guidelines, 2005) state that the candidates for biological therapy for psoriasis should have severe disease and fulfill at least one of the following criteria:[5]

A. Are or have become intolerant to or cannot receive standard therapy; or
B. Are or have become unresponsive to standard therapy; or
C. Have developed or are at higher than average risk of developing clinically important drug-related toxicity and where alternative standard therapy cannot be used; or
D. Have disease that is only controlled by repeated inpatient management; or
E. Have psoriatic arthritis fulfilling the British Society for Rheumatology (BSR) eligibility criteria for treatment with antitumor necrosis factor [TNF] agents, in association with skin disease; or
F. Have severe, unstable, life-threatening disease (erythrodermic or pustular psoriasis); or
G. Have significant, coexistant, unrelated comorbidity that precludes the use of systemic agents such as cyclosporine or methotrexate.

What is standard systemic therapy?

Standard systemic therapy has been defined to include acitretin, cyclosporine, methotrexate, narrow-band UVB, and PUVA, in British Association of Dermatology guidelines (BAD guidelines). According to these guidelines, a person is considered unresponsive to standard therapy if there is an unsatisfactory clinical response (a less than 50% improvement in baseline PASI score or precentage body surface area and less than 5% improvement in DLQI) to at least 3 months of treament in the therapeutic dose range of standard systemic therapy.[6]

Following dose ranges apply to the standard systemic therapy, according to BAD guidelines:

- Acitretin 25 to 50 mg daily
- Cyclosporine 2.5 to 5 mg per kg daily
- Methotrexate 15 mg, max 25 to 30 mg
- A maximum of 350 treatments for narrow band UVB and 150 to 200 treatments for PUVA (nonresponse, rapid relapse, or exceeding recommended maximum doses).

ALEFACEPT

Alefacept is a bivalent recombinant fusion protein which is composed of the first extracellular domain of lymphocyte function associated antigen 3 (LFA-3), fused to the hinge CH2 domain and CH3 domain of human IgG1. The LFA-3 portion of alefacept binds to CD2 receptors on T-cells, thereby blocking their natural interaction with LFA-3 on antigen presenting cells (APCs). The IgG1 portion of alefacept binds to FcγR receptor on natural killer cells to induce T-cell apoptosis. This cytotoxic effect is selective for the activated memory T-cells.[7] The US food and drug administration (FDA) has approved alefacept in January 2003 for treatment in adult patients with moderate to severe chronic plaque psoriasis, who are candidates for systemic therapy or phototherapy.

Mode of Administration[8,9]

Alefacept is given by intramuscular or intravenous route. The recommended dose of alefacept is 7.5 mg given once-weekly as an IV bolus or 15 mg given once-weekly as an IM injection. The recommended regimen is a course of 12 weekly injections. Retreatment with an additional 12-week course may be initiated provided that CD4+ T lymphocyte counts are within the normal range, and a minimum of a 12-week interval has passed since the previous course of treatment. Data on retreatment beyond 2 cycles are limited. The CD4+ T lymphocyte counts of patients receiving alefacept should be monitored weekly before initiating treatment and throughout the course of the 12-week dosing regimen. The treatment should be withheld if CD4+ T lymphocyte counts are below 250 cells/μL. The drug should be discontinued if the counts remain below 250 cells/μL for one month. The most frequently reported side-effects to alefacept include sore throat, dizziness, cough, headache, nausea, pruritus, muscle aches, chills, and pain and inflammation at the injection site. The most serious side-effects are lymphopenia, malignancies, serious infections and allergic reactions.

Evidence of Efficacy

Two 12-week courses of once-weekly intravenous alefacept 7.5 mg and placebo were given in a randomized double-blind study.[10] Patients were followed up for 12 weeks after each course. During treatment and follow-up of course 1, a 75% or greater reduction in the PASI was achieved by 28% of alefacept treated and 8% of placebo-treated patients ($p < 0.001$). Patients who received a single course of alefacept and achieved a 75% or greater reduction from baseline PASI during or after treatment (without the use of phototherapy or systemic therapies), maintained a 50% or greater reduction in PASI for a median duration of more than 7 months. Among patients who received 2 courses of alefacept, 40% and 71% of patients achieved a 75% or greater and 50% or greater reduction in PASI, respectively, during the study period. Alefacept was well-tolerated over both courses. In an international, randomized, double-blind, placebo-controlled, parallel-group trial with total of 507 patients with chronic plaque psoriasis, patients were administered either 10 mg of alefacept or 15 mg of alefacept once-weekly for 12 weeks, followed by 12 weeks of observation. In the 15 mg group, 33% patients achieved 75% reduction in PASI, 2 weeks after the last dose and 71% maintained at least 50% improvement in PASI throughout the 12-week follow-up. Comparatively, 28% patients achieved 75% reduction in PASI in the 10 mg group[11] (thus higher dose was more effective).

EFALIZUMAB

Efalizumab is a recombinant humanized monoclonal IgG1 antibody that binds to CD11a, the α subunit of leukocyte function-associated antigen 1 (LFA-1). It disrupts the interaction between LFA-1 and intercellular adhesion molecules (ICAM-1, a ligand of LFA-1), a cell surface molecule expressed by antigen presenting cells (APCs). ICAM-1 is up-regulated on both endothelial cells and keratinocytes within psoriatic plaques.[12] The effects of efalizumab are confined only to those cells expressing LFA-1. It has been suggested that efalizumab destabilizes the binding of APCs and T-cells and thereby reduces the efficiency of initial T-cell activation in lymph nodes. It also decreases the trafficking of T-cells from the circulation into dermal and epidermal tissues and interferes with the secondary activation of memory-effector T-cells in the target tissues. Efalizumab was approved by the US FDA in October 2003 for the treatment of psoriasis. It is currently the only biologic agent approved for continuous administration to adult patients.[13]

Mode of Administration

Efalizumab is given as subcutaneous injection, with patients being instructed to rotate the injection sites between the thigh, abdomen, buttocks and upper arm with each dose. The recommended dose of efalizumab is 1 mg/kg weekly as a subcutaneous, self-administered injection for 12 weeks, following an induction dose of 0.7 mg/kg, with the recommendation that treatment should be continued only in those who respond.[14] No single dose should exceed 200 mg. A single use vial of efalizumab contains 125 mg of drug as sterile lyophilized powder, with preloaded single use syringes containing 1.3 mL of sterile water. Acute flu-like symptoms including headache, chills, fever, nausea and myalgia may occur within 48 hours after administration of the first two doses. A complete blood count including platelet count should be done at the start of therapy and repeated periodically while the patient is on treatment. Autoimmune hemolytic anemia may occur 4–6 months after the start of treatment with efalizumab. The drug should be discontinued if thrombocytopenia or hemolytic anemia occurs. Concurrent immunosuppressive therapy should be avoided.[15]

Evidence of Efficacy

The safety and efficacy of efalizumab has been evaluated in four large phase III studies in 2000 patients with moderate-to-severe chronic plaque psoriasis, most of whom had unsuccessfully received previous systemic therapy for psoriasis.[16-19] Efalizumab appeared to be effective, with 27% of patients who received a dose of 1 mg/kg weekly, achieved PASI 75 (>75% reduction in baseline PASI score) compared to 4% in placebo group by week 12. Continuation of therapy beyond 12 weeks has been found to increase the response rate further. The relapse of psoriasis has been reported to occur approximately about 2 months of discontinuation of therapy and rebound in approximately 5% of the patients, as defined by flaring >125% of baseline.

ETANERCEPT

Etanercept is a recombinant fully human dimeric fusion protein (human TNF-α p75 receptor and the Fc portion of human IgG1 molecule fused together) which acts as a TNF inhibitor by binding to and inactivating TNF-α, thereby preventing interaction with its cell surface receptors on target cells and blocking its proinflammatory effects.[20] Etanercept is FDA approved for use in adults with moderate-to-severe psoriasis, who are candidates for systemic therapy or phototherapy. The drug is also indicated for treatment of psoriatic arthritis, rheumatoid arthritis (including juvenile rheumatoid arthritis) and ankylosing spondylitis.[21,22] Etanercept is available in India among the biological for psoriasis (Wyeth Ltd, Worli, Mumbai). It is available as 25 mg dose per vial as a sterile, white, preservative free lyophilized powder for parenteral administration, after reconstitution with 1 mL of the supplied sterile bacteriostatic water for injection.

Mode of Administration

Etanercept is given as injection by subcutaneous route. The adult dose is 50 mg/week, given subcutaneously usually for 12–24 weeks. It can be self-administered by the patient and the most common site for these injections are the abdomen, thighs and upper arms.[23] The most frequent side-effects of etanercept include mild, transient injection site reactions, upper respiratory tract infections, headache and rhinitis.

Evidence of Efficacy

The available current literature recommends use of intermittent courses of subcutaneous injections of etanercept up to a maximum of 24 weeks.[24] Several small phase II studies and two key phase III randomized controlled trials involving about 1,000 patients with moderate- to-severe chronic plaque psoriasis (in whom previous systemic treatment and phototherapy had been ineffective), indicate that etanercept is an effective treatment for chronic plaque psoriasis. Efficacy is dose-related, with 34% of patients receiving 25 mg and 49% receiving 50 mg twice weekly, achieving PASI 75 after 12 weeks of treatment (thus higher dose is more effective). The time to relapse after a complete course (after 24 weeks of therapy), ranged from 70–91 days and appeared to be dose-related, i.e. remission is maintained longer in higher dose group as compared to the lower dose group. Of patients achieving PASI 75 response at 24 weeks of therapy, 11% remained in remission for 1 year.[25,26]

INFLIXIMAB

Infliximab is a human-mouse monoclonal anti-TNF-α antibody[27] that binds with high affinity to both soluble and transmembrane-bound forms of TNF-α and inhibits the ability of TNF-α to bind with its receptors. Infliximab also indirectly inhibits production of other proinflammatory cytokines. A significant decrease in cytokines IL-6, VEGF, FGF and E-selectin has been detected after infliximab infusions. It is also suggested that the binding of infliximab to membrane-bound TNF-α results in lysis of TNF-α producing cells by means of a complement or antibody dependent cell-mediated cytotoxic mechanism.[27] Infliximab is approved for the treatment of Crohn's disease and rheumatoid arthritis. It is effective in the treatment of moderate to severe psoriasis and psoriatic arthritis. Infliximab may also be of value in recalcitrant or unstable disease and in generalized pustular psoriasis.[28] Low dose infliximab has also been used in combination with methotrexate in severe recalcitrant psoriasis.

Mode of Administration

Infliximab is given as an intravenous infusion in doses of 5–10 mg/kg over a period of 2 hours at weeks 0, 2 and 6 and may be followed by repeat single infusions at 8–12 week intervals.[29] The side-effects which are usually seen with infliximab infusion include infections, headache, vertigo, flushing, gastrointestinal effects, abnormal hepatic functions and fatigue.

Evidence of Efficacy

In two randomized placebo-controlled trials,[30-32] in patients with moderate to severe stable chronic plaque psoriasis, 75% improvement in PASI scores at week 10 were noted in 87% of patients receiving standard induction course of therapy, with significant improvement in the quality of life. Time to relapse following successful induction therapy was highly variable between individuals and was noted to depend on the initial dose given, with 73% of those given 10 mg/kg during induction maintained at least 50% improvement in PASI scores at week 26, compared to 40% of those given 5 mg/kg.

ADALIMUMAB

Adalimumab is a human IgG1 monoclonal anti-TNF-α antibody directed against TNF-α and blocks its interaction with the p55 and p75 cell surface receptors. It also lyses the cells that express surface TNF-α in the presence of complement. Currently, the drug is undergoing phase-II clinical trials for psoriasis and phase III studies for psoriatic arthritis.[33] Adalimumab is FDA approved for the treatment of rheumatoid arthritis, in a dose of 40 mg subcutaneously every other week and is undergoing clinical trials (phase III) for the treatment of psoriatic arthritis. In a double-blind, randomized, placebo-controlled trial,[34] patients with moderate-to-severe active psoriatic arthritis and a history of inadequate response to nonsteroidal antiinflammatory drugs were randomized to receive 40 mg adalimumab or placebo subcutaneously, every other week for 24 weeks. The patients were followed up at weeks 2 and 4 and every 4 weeks thereafter. Adalimumab was found to be safe and well-tolerated, improved joint and skin manifestations significantly, prevented progression of structural changes on radiographs, decreased disability due to joint damage and brought improved quality of life in patients with moderate-to-severe active psoriatic arthritis.

BRODALUMAB, SECUKINUMAB

Anti IL-17. It is being tested for the treatment of moderate-to-severe psoriasis and is in phase III clinical trials. Secukinumab is a human monoclonal antibody designed for the treatment of uveitis, rheumatoid arthritis and psoriasis. It has completed phase III clinical trials for plaque psoriasis in 2011.[35]

USTEKINUMAB

Ustekinumab is a fully human monoclonal antibody that binds with high specificity and affinity to the cytokines interleukin IL-12 and IL-23, thereby suppressing IL-12 and IL-23-mediated inflammation associated with psoriasis. Ustekinumab was approved for the treatment of adults with moderate-to-severe psoriasis in September 2009 by US FDA alone or in combination with methotrexate for the treatment of adult patients with active psoriatic arthritis.

Mode of Injection—Subcutaneous

For the treatment of psoriatic arthritis, ustekinumab is administered as a 45 mg subcutaneous injection at weeks 0 and 4, and then every 12 weeks, thereafter. For patients with coexistent moderate-to-severe plaque psoriasis weighing more than 220 lbs (100 kg) the recommended dose is 90 mg subcutaneous injection at weeks 0 and 4, and then every 12 weeks, thereafter.[36]

GOLIMUMAB AND CERTOLIZUMAB PEGOL

Anti-TNF alpha. Golimumab is approved in Canada and United States as a once monthly subcutaneous treatment for adults with moderate-to-severly active rheumatoid arthritis, psoriatic arthritis and ankylosing spondylitis. On September 2013, the US FDA approved Certolizumab for use in United States for the treatment of adult patients with active psoriatic arthritis.[37]

OTHER BIOLOGICAL AGENTS

Onercept a recombinant human soluble p55 tumor necrosis factor binding protein which is being tested for its efficacy in psoriasis.

Fezakinumab targets IL-22 cytokine and is in trial phase for the treatment of psoriasis.

OKTcdr4a, CTLA-41g, Denileukin diftitox; Basiliximab and Daclizumab ab (anti CD25), **Siplizumab** (anti CD2) are in trial phase for psoriasis.[38]

Points to Remember

- Biologicals are a recent addition to the therapeutic armamentarium of psoriasis. The biologics, because of their specific action on the immune system, have very little side-effects
- The British Association of Dermatologists (2005) stated that candidates for biological therapies for psoriasis should have severe disease and fulfill at least one of the following criteria:
  - Are or have become intolerant to or cannot receive standard therapy; or
  - Are or have become unresponsive to standard therapy; or
  - Have developed or are at higher than average risk of developing clinically important drug-related toxicity and where alternative standard therapy cannot be used; or
  - Have disease that is only controlled by repeated inpatient management; or
  - Have psoriatic arthritis fulfilling the British Society for Rheumatology (BSR) eligibility criteria for treatment with anti-tumor necrosis factor [TNF] agents, in association with skin disease; or
  - Have severe, unstable, life-threatening disease (erythrodermic or pustular psoriasis); or
  - Have significant, coexistant, unrelated comorbidity that precludes the use of systemic agents such as cyclosporine or methotrexate.

REFERENCES

1. Parrish JA, Stern RS, Pathak MA, Fitzpatrick TB. Photochemotherapy of skin disease. In: Regan JD, Parrish JA, (Eds). The science of photomedicine. New York: Plenum Press; 1982:595-623.
2. Bansback N, Sizto S, Sun H, et al. Efficacy of systemic treatments for moderate-to-severe plaque psoriasis: Systematic review and meta-analysis. Dermatology. 2009;219(3):209-18.
3. Tzu J, Krulig E, Cardenas V, Kerdel FA. Biological agents in the treatment of psoriasis. G Ital Dermatol Venereol. 2008;143(5):315-27.
4. Finnish Medical Society Duodecim. Psoriasis. In: EBM Guidelines. Evidence-Based Medicine [CD-ROM]. Helsinki, Finland: Duodecim Medical Publications Ltd. 2005.
5. British Association of Dermatologists (BAD). Psoriasis Guideline London, UK: BAD; 2006.
6. Smith CH, Anstey JNWN, Barker AD, et al. British Association of Dermatologists guidelines for use of biological interventions in psoriasis 2005. Br J Dermatol. 2005;153:486-97.
7. Krueger GG. Current concepts and review of alefacept in the treatment of psoriasis. Dermatol Clin 2004;22:407-26.
8. Kormeili T, Lowe NJ, Yamuchi PS. Psoriasis: Immunopathogenesis and evolving immunomodulators and systemic therapies; US experiences. Br J Dermatol 2004;151:3-15.
9. Krueger GG, Papp KA, Stough DB, Loven KH, Gulliver WP, Ellis CN. Alefacept Clinical Study Group. A randomized, double-blind, placebo-controlled phase III study evaluating efficacy and tolerability of 2 courses of alefacept in patients with chronic plaque psoriasis. J Am Acad Dermatol 2002;47:821-33.
10. Lebwohl M, Christophers E, Langley R, Ortonne JP, Roberts J, Griffiths CE, et al. Alefacept clinical study group. An international, randomized, double-blind, placebo-controlled phase 3 trial of intramuscular alefacept in patients with chronic plaque psoriasis. Arch Dermatol 2003;139:719-27.
11. Menter A, Cather JC, Baker D, Farber HF, Lebwohi M, Darif M. The efficacy of multiple courses of alefacept in patients with moderate-to-severe chronic plaque psoriasis. J Am Acad Dermatol 2006;54:61-3.
12. Leonardi CL. Current concepts and review of efalizumab in the treatment of psoriasis. Dermatol Clin 2004;22:427-35.
13. Lebwohl M, Tyring SK, Hamilton TK, Toth D, Glazer S, Tawfik NH, et al. A novel targeted T-cell modulator, efalizumab, for plaque psoriasis. N Engl J Med 2003;21:2004-13.
14. Gordon KB, Papp KA, Hamilton TK, Walicke PA, Dummer W, Li N, et al. Efalizumab for patients with moderate to severe plaque psoriasis: A randomized control trial. JAMA 2003;23:3073-80.
15. Joshi R. Immunopathogenesis of psoriasis. Indian J Dermatol Venerol Leprol 2004;70:10-2.

16. Leonardi CL, Papp KA, Gordon KB, Menter A, Feldman SR, Caro I, et al. Extended efalizumab therapy improves chronic plaque psoriasis: Results from a randomized phase III trials. J Am Acad Dermatol 2005; 52:425-33.
17. Menter A, Gordon K, Carey W, Hamilton T, Glazer S, Caro I, et al. Efficacy and safety observed during 24 weeks of efalizumab therapy in patients with moderate to severe plaque psoriasis. Arch Dermatol 2005;141:31-8.
18. Brimhall AK, King LN, Licciardone JC, et al. Safety and efficacy of alefacept, efalizumab, etanercept and infliximab in treating moderate to severe plaque psoriasis: A meta-analysis of randomized controlled trials. Br J Dermatol. 2008; 159(2):274-85.
19. Boudreau R, Blackhouse G, Goeree R, Mierzwinski-Urban M. Adalimumab, elefacept, efalizumab, etanercept, and infliximab for severe psoriasis vulgaris in adults: Budget impact analysis and review of comparative clinical- and cost-effectiveness. Technology Report No. 97. Ottawa, ON: Canadian Agency for Drugs and Technologies in Health (CADTH); 2007.
20. Smith CH, Anstey AV, Barker JN, Burden AD, Chalmers RJ, Chandler D, et al. British association of Dermatologists guidelines for use of biological interventions in psoriasis 2005. Br J Dermatol 2005;153:486-97.
21. Goldsmith DR, Wagstaff AJ. Etanercept: A review of its use in the management of plaque psoriasis and psoriatic arthritis. Am J Clin Dermatol 2005;6:121-36.
22. Yamuchi PS, Gindi V, Lowe NJ. The treatment of psoriasis and psoriatic arthritis with etanercept: Practical considerations on monotherapy, combination therapy and safety. Dermatol Clin 2004;22:449-59.
23. Kormeili T, Lowe NJ, Yamuchi PS. Psoriasis: Immunopathogenesis and evolving immunomodulators and systemic therapies; US experiences. Br J Dermatol 2004;151:3-15.
24. Smith CH, Anstey AV, Barker JN, Burden AD, Chalmers RJ, Chandler D, et al. British association of Dermatologists guidelines for use of biological interventions in psoriasis 2005. Br J Dermatol 2005;153:486-97.
25. Gottlieb AB, Matheson RT, Lowe N, Krueger GG, Kang S, Goffe BS, et al. A randomized trial of etanercept as monotherapy for psoriasis. Arch Dermatol 2003;139:1627-32.
26. Leonardi CL, Powers JL, Matheson RT, Goffe BS, Zitnik R, Wang A, et al. Etanercept as monotherapy in patients with psoriasis. N Engl J Med 2003;349:2014-22.
27. Papp KA, Tyring S, Lahfa M, Prinz J, Griffiths CE, Nakanishi AM, et al. A global Phase III randomized control trial of etanercept in psoriasis: Safety, efficacy and effect of dose reduction. Br J Dermatol 2005;152:1304-12.
28. Winterfield L, Menter A. Psoriasis and its treatment with infliximab-mediated tumour necrosis factor a blockade. Dermatol Clin 2004;22:437-44.
29. Mastroianni A, Minutilli E, Mussi A, Bordignon V. Cytokine profiles during infliximab monotherapy in psoriatic arthritis. Br J Dermatol 2005;153:531-6.
30. Chaudhari U, Romano P, Mulcahy LD, Dooley LT, Baker DG, Gottlieb AB. Efficacy and safety of infliximab montherapy for plaque type psoriasis: A randomized trial. Lancet 2001;35:1842-7.
31. Gottlieb AB, Evans R, Li S, Dooley LT, Guzzo CA, Baker D. Infliximab induction therapy for patients with severe plaque type psoriasis: A randomized, double-blind, placebo controlled trial. J Am Acad Dermatol 2004;51:534-42.
32. Zargari O. Sustained effects of low dose infliximab in combination with methotrexate in the management of chronic recalcitrant psoriasis. Dermatol Online J 2005;11:21.
33. Scheinfeld N. Adalimumab (HUMIRA): A review. J Drugs Dermatol 2003;2:375-7.
34. Mease PJ, Gladman DD, Ritchlin CT, Ruderman EM, Steinfeld SD, Choy EH, et al. Adalimumab for the treatment of patients with moderately-to-severely active psoriatic arthritis: Results of a double-blind, randomized, placebo-controlled trial. Arthritis Rheum 2005;52:3279-89.
35. Sterry W, Barker J, Boehncke WH, Bos JD, Chimenti S, Christophers E, et al. Biological therapies in the systemic management of psoriasis: International Consensus Conference. Br J Dermatol. 2004;151: 69:3-17.
36. Gottlieb AB, Menter A, Mendelsohn A, et al. Ustekinumab, a human interleukin 12/23 monoclonal antibody for psoriatic arthritis: a randomised, double-blind placebo-controlled, crossover trial. Lancet 2009;373: 633-40.
37. Hutas G. Golimumab, a fully human monoclonal antibody against TNF alpha. Curr Opin Mol Ther. 2008;10: 393-406.
38. Rozenblit M, Lebwohl M. New biologics for psoriasis and psoriatic arthritis. Dermatol Ther. 2009;22(1):56-60.

Chapter

42

Ambulatory Treatment (Day Care) for Psoriasis

Ambulatory care or outpatient care is medical care provided on an outpatient basis, including diagnosis, observation, consultation, treatment, intervention and rehabilitation services. The advantages of this care are quicker recovery without having to hospitalize the patient and greater patient freedom during the treatment. Ambulatory treatment centers in case of psoriasis provide specialized combination therapies such as Goeckerman and Ingram's regimen, in addition to standard office treatments for psoriasis. Traditional treatment plans may vary depending on the individual center and they allow for extended periods of care under the supervision of a physician. Additional services in psoriasis which are provided in day care centers may include specialized scalp treatments such as PUVA turban therapy, nail treatment, patient education sessions and psychological support groups.

Before considering specific treatment in an individual psoriatic patient, it is important to exclude aggravating factors such as infections, steroid intake/withdrawal, use of medications containing heavy metals and psychological stress. The area of involvement, impairment of the quality of life and responsiveness to previous treatments has to be taken into account.

Approximately, 20% of psoriasis patients require systemic therapy to improve their skin condition. Phototherapy with UVB or PUVA (Psoralens plus Ultraviolet A) is often the next recommended choice of treatment. Proper patient selection and pretreatment assessment, good dosimetry and protocol and regular monitoring will result in a good therapeutic index.

Goeckerman therapy, first formulated in 1925 by American dermatologist William H Goeckerman is a regimen used for the treatment of moderate-to-severe plaque psoriasis in which 2–4% crude coal tar in a petrolatum base is applied daily to the psoriatic plaques. The minimum period of time for tar application is 2 hours, although larger periods of application have been observed to better results. The patient is then exposed to broad-band or narrow-band UVB.

The Ingram regimen combines anthralin paste and UVB exposure. Anthralin is applied to lesions as a thick paste. Once anthralin is removed, the patient is then exposed to UVB and may also take coal tar baths. Generally, a patient using the ingram regimen in a day care center will require approximately 3 weeks for clearance.

SUGGESTED READINGS

1. Larko O, Swanbeck G. Psoriasis treatment and a day care center: Clinical aspects and an attempt at cost benefit analysis. Acta Derm Venereol. 1982;62:413-18.

Chapter

43 Indications for Hospitalization in Psoriasis

Psoriasis is usually managed on an outpatient basis. However, some patients may require inpatient treatment or hospitalization. The criteria for admission may include the following:

i. Acute erythrodermic psoriasis: It is characterized by involvement of >90% of the body surface area. The persistent and universal inflammation of the skin associated with erythroderma has important consequences for thermoregulation, hemodynamics, protein and water metabolism. It can be associated with appreciable mortality and hence needs hospitalization and appropriate management.

ii. Acute generalized pustular psoriasis: It is a severe form of psoriasis which can be precipitated by infections, hypocalcemia, antimalarials, tar and withdrawal of corticosteroids. Generalized pustular psoriasis can revert to an erythrodermic state with its attendant complications. Topical treatments are usually avoided in pustular psoriasis and hospitalization is recommended in acute generalized pustular psoriasis.

iii. Hyperacute psoriatic polyarthritis that threatens irreversible joint damage. Distal interphalangeal joint involvement and oligoarthritis is characteristically seen in psoriasis. However, rheumatoid like polyarthritis, involvement of axial skeleton and mutilating arthritis need a multidisciplinary approach and appropriate management.

iv. Psoriasis not controlled with outpatient treatment. This subgroup of patients is usually associated with psychological stress which forms a vicious circle with excess smoking and alcohol intake, and hence exacerbation of the disease.

v. Complications from previous treatment such as topical, systemic, phototherapy or photochemotherapy, and not controlled with outpatient therapy. In this subgroup of patients, psoriatic erythroderma or pustular psoriasis is usually seen which forms a mandatory indication for hospitalization.

vi. Psoriasis that is physically or emotionally disabling enough to limit activities of daily living. The psychosocial impact of the disease is associated with increased stress, which forms a vicious circle, thus leading to an exacerbation of the disease.

ADJUNCTIVE THERAPIES FOR PSORIASIS

Adjunctive therapies for psoriasis consist of:

i. Antihistamines/Antibiotics.
ii. Occlusive dressings and/or suits.
iii. Wet dressings.
iv. Antifungal creams/Antibacterial creams.
v. Specialized baths.
vi. Psychiatric counseling.

INDICATIONS OF REFERRAL TO A DERMATOLOGIST IN CASE OF PSORIASIS

The patients with psoriasis need to be referred to a specialist dermatologist in case of the following:

- If there is diagnostic uncertainty
- Any type of psoriasis that is extensive or severe enough (PASI>10%, BSA>10%)
- Failure of topical therapy to control psoriasis
- Psoriatic arthritis
- Generalized pustular psoriasis
- Psoriatic erythroderma
- Any type of psoriasis that has a major impact on the patient's physical, psychological and social wellbeing
- Childhood psoriasis.

SUGGESTED READINGS

1. NICE Guidelines (2012). Psoriasis. The assessment and management of psoriasis.
2. The British Associations of Dermatologists (2006). General management of psoriasis—Recommendations.

Chapter

44 Counselling and Patient Education in Psoriasis

Psoriasis has a detrimental effect on the psychosocial quality of life of patients, which is almost similar to that of major diseases such as heart disease. There is ample evidence for the role of stress in the onset and aggravation of psoriasis. Various studies have shown that stress management programs significantly decrease the time to clearance when used in conjunction with standard therapies. Increased stress is associated with excess alcohol intake and smoking, both of which are known aggravating factors for psoriasis. Hence, counseling and patient education form an important part of any treatment plan and should include information on the disease and the effects that trauma, alcohol, infection and stress may have on psoriasis. Expectations of the results of therapy and interactions that are possible between phototherapy and drugs and the disease are to be considered as part of the patient education. It is very important for patients to be partners in treatment.[1] At diagnosis the following should be provided:

i. Booklet on psoriasis: Booklet will provide all the basic information about the disease, including the exacerbating factors.
ii. Counseling to patients and/or relatives, regarding the various treatment modalities available for the disease and the minimal effect of the disease on the quality of life when managed appropriately and avoiding the exacerbating factors, such as stress, smoking and alcohol.
iii. Patients should be taught on side-effects, possible provoking factors and warned on harmful treatments.

REFERENCE

1. Parisi R, Symmons DPM, Griffiths CEM, Ashcroft DM. The identification and management of psoriasis and associated comorbidity project team. Global epidemiology of psoriasis: a systematic review of incidence and prevalence. Journal of Investigative Dermatology. 2013;133:377-85.

Chapter 45

Complimentary Therapies for Psoriasis

Various complimentary/nonpharmacological therapies have been tried in psoriasis from times immemorial. These are used in addition to the standard therapeutic modalities for the management of psoriasis. An attempt has been made to briefly discuss various complimentary therapies for psoriasis in this chapter.

Various complimentary therapies for psoriasis are:

1. *Climatotherapy:* Refers to temporary or permanent relocation of a patient to a region with a climate more favorable to recovery from or management of a condition. Examples include:
   - Since the partial pressure of oxygen is lower at high altitude, so person with sickle cell disease might move to a lower altitude to reduce the number of sickle crises
   - Several sites around the world are advertised or studied as possibly of therapeutic benefit to patients with psoriasis, most notably the Dead Sea region

   Exposure to sunlight and Dead Sea water bathing are considered to be most important. In a study by Even-Paz et al., it was observed that the major therapeutic factor is exposure to sunlight, whereas Dead Sea water only enhances the effect of the sun. The recommendations for Climatotherapy at the Dead Sea (CDS) consist of sunlight exposure at a maximum of 3 hours daily in the spring and summer, divided into morning and afternoon sessions. Climatotherapy at the Dead Sea (CDS) for patients with psoriasis induces a persistent remission in the majority of patients with psoriasis, is associated with minor side-effects and is pleasant for the patients. The published literature on CDS describes patients with moderate-to-severe psoriasis who spend an average period of one month (long-term) at the Dead Sea. There are no published data, however, on the effectiveness and characteristics of short-term CDS for patients with psoriasis, who spend only 2 weeks at the Dead Sea.
2. *Thalassotherapy:* Thalassotherapy (from the Greek word thalassa, meaning "sea") involves ocean-based treatments, which often utilize seaweed, salt water and marine mud. While people have recognized the healing power of the ocean waters for thousands of years, thalassotherapy was developed in the seaside towns of France during the 1800's to take advantage of these benefits. Today, common treatments offered at spas include seawater baths, marine mud baths, seaweed wraps and massages. Thalassotherapy takes advantage of the minerals found in seawater, seaweed and marine mud, including magnesium, potassium, calcium, sodium and iodine. Theses minerals have been shown to be beneficial to the skin and a person's general health and wellbeing. The salt water soothes dry skin and fights psoriasis, eczema and acne.
3. *Balneotherapy:* Is defined as the use of baths containing thermal mineral waters from natural springs at a temperature of at least 20°C and with a mineral content of at least 1 g/L. More so, it is more common that the temperature of the thermal water is approximately

34°C. Balneotherapy has been used not only in the ancient years in the treatment of various illnesses but also in modern times.

Under the broad term balneotherapy (in contrast to the strict definition given above), various treatment methods are included: Dead Sea salt or mineral baths, sulfur baths and radon-carbon dioxide baths. Balneotherapy is either provided as the solitary component of the therapeutic approach or in the context of spa therapy. Spa therapy additionally to balneotherapy employs various modalities such as physiotherapy and even the change in environment and lifestyle *per se* may contribute to the changes seen in patient outcome measurements, i.e. the therapeutic result may not be attributed to the balneotherapy alone. Thus, while some researchers have regarded balneotherapy and spas as more or less interchangeable terms, others disagree.

ICHTHYOTHERAPY IN PSORIASIS

Ichthyotherapy (therapy with the so-called 'Doctor fish of Kangal', Garra rufa) has been shown to be effective in patients with psoriasis in the Kangal hot springs in Turkey. Several mechanisms have been suggested regarding the observed efficacy of ichthyotherapy in Turkey. One obvious mechanism is the physical contact with the fish, which feed on the desquamating skin, thus leading to a rapid reduction of the scales. Another suggested mechanism is the direct effect of natural UV radiation owing to the high altitude (1650 m) of the Kangal spa. Phototherapy is a well-recognized option for patients with widespread psoriasis, lesions with climatotherapy being the simplest form. However, a simultaneous removal of scales by the fish probably facilitates the penetration of UV rays into the dermis. This exposure of the lesions may explain the better outcome of combined ichthyotherapy/UVA treatment when compared with the poor results of UVA sunbed treatment alone. A third suggested mechanism of ichthyotherapy in Kangal is the presence of a high level of selenium (1.3 mg/L) in the hot spring water. A fourth mechanism suggested by Ozcelik et al. is the reverse Koebner phenomenon. The reverse Koebner phenomenon is seen when an area of psoriasis clears following injury.

HYDROTHERAPY (WATER THERAPY)

Water therapy as practiced today was introduced in Austria in the 19th century by Father Sebastian Kneipp. Father Kneipp believed in the healing properties of water and prescribed treatments that included drinking mineral waters, soaking in hot springs, taking cold showers, and walking barefoot in the early-morning dew. Healing spas that adhered to Father Kneipp's philosophy sprang up all over Europe and "taking the waters" became a popular social pastime for the rich and privileged.

HERBAL REMEDIES

Herbal remedies use substances derived from plants to treat the patient's condition. In the case of psoriasis, this can vary from topical treatments such as *aloe vera, orgeon grape root cream and neem oil,* to medicines that are taken orally.

There are entire systems of herbal therapy that can be followed, such as *traditional chinese medicine, western herbal medicine* and *ayurvedic medicine,* which often also incorporate elements of spiritualism and diet into the therapy. However, extreme care must be taken when using these substances, especially if the label is not in English. The MHRA has investigated reports into the use of mercury, lead and arsenic in unlicensed *ayurvedic* and *traditional* Chinese medicines and some patients in the USA have recently suffered lead poisoning after taking certain *ayurvedic* remedies.

Again, it is important to look for a THR number on all herbal remedies, as this proves that the product is registered with the MHRA and has achieved UK standards of quality and safety.

HOMEOPATHIC REMEDIES

Homeopathic is a system that aims to stimulate the body's natural defences. The practitioner will treat 'like with like', using very diluted doses of substances that are believed to cause similar symptoms when taken in higher doses. Again, these are often 'natural' products (although they may not originate from plants), such as sulfur, nickel and silica.

Homeopathic treatment should be tailored to each patient, and therefore should involve consultation with a licensed practitioner, who can ensure that the substances are diluted and measured enough to be safe. The detailed discussion is beyond the scope of this book.

MIND/BODY THERAPIES

Research has looked at links between psoriasis and psychological factors such as stress and emotions. It is recognized that stress can trigger or worsen psoriasis in some people. There is, therefore, a school of thought that relaxing the mind could help to abate the condition of the body. Therapies that teach relaxation and stress reduction techniques include *counseling, cognitive behaviour therapy, meditation, aromatherapy, floatation and hypnotherapy.*

PHYSICAL THERAPIES

These involve the physical manipulation of the body through techniques such as massage, acupuncture or acupressure, chiropractic and osteopathy. Massage and acupuncture/pressure are often used as relaxation therapies, to release tension in certain areas of the body. Chiropractic and osteopathy, however, are primary healthcare professions that use physical manipulation to increase joint mobility, relieve pain and muscle spasm and enhance blood supply. These may be particularly helpful to patients with psoriatic arthritis.

Points to Remember

The use of complimentary therapies such as climatotherapy, ichthyotherapy and balneotherapy should be considered in addition to the routine treatment to increase the duration of remission and improve the quality of life in patients with psoriasis

SUGGESTED READINGS

1. Schenidman HM. Treatment of psoriasis at the dead Sea. In: Epstein E (Ed). Controversies in dermatology. Philadelphia: WB Saunders. 1984:243-46.

Chapter

46 Diet and Nutrition in Psoriasis

Psoriasis is considered as a T-cell-mediated inflammatory skin disease which is characterized by hyperproliferation and poor differentiation of epidermal keratinocytes. While susceptibility to psoriasis is inherited, the disease is influenced by environmental factors such as infections and stress. Diet has been suggested to play a role in the etiology and pathogenesis of psoriasis. Various dietary modifications have/and are being tried in psoriatic patients, but have been found to make no appreciable difference in the course of the disease. Intermittent periods of fasting, low-energy diets, intake of fresh fruits and vegetables have been found to improve psoriasis in some studies and diets rich in ω-3 polyunsaturated fatty acids from fish oil have also show beneficial effects on the course of psoriasis. All these diets modify the polyunsaturated fatty acid metabolism and influence the eicosanoid profile, so that inflammatory processes are suppressed. Some patients with psoriasis show an elevated sensitivity to gluten. In patients with IgA and/or IgG antigliadin antibodies, the symptoms have been shown to improve on a gluten-free diet. The active form of vitamin D (1,25-dihydroxyvitamin D_3), exhibits antiproliferative and immunoregulatory effects via the vitamin D receptor, and thus is responsible for the beneficial effect of vitamin-D analogues in the topical treatment of psoriasis. In this chapter, an attempt is made to discuss the role of dietary factors in psoriasis.

The dietary factors that may play a role in psoriasis are as follows:[1-3]

1. *Dietary intake:* The prevalence and severity of psoriasis have been reported to be lower during the periods of fasting and fasting has been found to improve psoriasis in few patients. Therefore, the disease may be improved by low-calorie diets. Psoriasis also has a positive correlation with obesity, i.e. more severely affected patients with psoriasis are more likely to be obese and hence, weight reduction is recommended in obese psoriatic patients. Obesity as a component of metabolic syndrome is now a well-defined associated causative/aggravating factor and the point of intervention for psoriasis. The link between psoriasis, obesity, hypertension, dyslipidemia and insulin resistance, better known as metabolic syndrome is responsible for the higher risk of myocardial infarction seen among relatively young, severely affected psoriatic patients. Similar cytokines (i.e. Th1) have been found in both psoriasis and obesity, which are responsible for the systemic inflammation, and hence the consequences of metabolic syndrome. Hence, weight reduction and regular exercise should be encouraged in patients with psoriasis.
2. *Smoking and alcohol:* Both smoking and alcohol have been suspected to have a negative impact on the severity of psoriasis from times immemorial. Smoking has been demonstrated to have a role in the onset of psoriasis in few studies, while other studies have found that

the prevalence of psoriasis in a population of individuals who stop smoking or who lose weight to decrease. More striking is the association between smoking and palmoplantar pustular psoriasis. Increased alcohol consumption is a recognized stress response. Alcohol stimulates histamine release and may therefore, aggravate skin lesions. The intake of alcohol is usually associated with obesity and concomitant increase in the intake of fatty foods and reduced consumption of fresh fruits and vegetables. Excess alcohol intake has been found to lead to treatment resistance and reduced therapeutic compliance. Hence, alcohol intake should be restricted in patients with psoriasis.

3. *Role of polyunsaturated fatty acids:* A number of uncontrolled studies have shown the beneficial effect of fish and fish oil supplementation (rich in ω-3 PUFAs) on psoriasis and psoriatic arthritis. The main constituents of fish oil are eicosapentaenoic acid (EPA) and docosahexaenoic acid (DHA). The basis for the anti-inflammatory effect of fish oil supplementation is the replacement of proinflammatory arachidonic acid in membrane phospholipids by anti-inflammatory ω-3 PUFAs [eicosapentaenoic acid (EPA) and DHA].[3]
4. *Role of gluten:* Various studies have established a causal relationship between celiac disease and gluten intake. Few studies have shown that there may be an increased incidence of psoriasis in patients with celiac disease. Patients with psoriasis have been found to have an increased incidence of IgG/IgA antigliadin antibodies (16% in one Sweden study) compared with healthy controls and a Sweden study has also demonstrated that a gluten free diet for a period of 3 months, especially in patients with antigliadin antibodies, improved disease severity in patients with psoriasis. The postulated mechanisms for worsening of psoriasis with gluten intake are:
   a. Gluten intake results in increased intestinal permeability in patients with latent gluten sensitivity, which can allow the passage of microbes that in turn act as superantigens and hence worsen psoriasis (infectious induced).
   b. Type-II inflammatory cytokines (IL-2, IFN-γ, TNF-α) has been demonstrated in psoriasis and celiac disease, which may be antigliadin antibody induced.
5. *Role of oxidative stress and antioxidants:* Various studies have shown the presence of oxidative stress and the resultant increase in free-radical generation to play a role in the inflammatory mechanism of psoriasis. The consumption of fresh fruits and vegetables, such as carrots and tomatoes, may be beneficial in psoriasis because of their high content of carotenoids, flavonoids and vitamin C. A sufficient intake of antioxidants (e.g. vitamin C, vitamin E, β-carotene and selenium) may be helpful to prevent an imbalance of oxidative stress and antioxidant defence in psoriasis.
6. *General dietary modifications:* Psoriatic erythroderma and extensive plaque psoriasis is well known to result in loss of proteins and other nutrients through scales, hence causing hypoproteinemia and nutritional deficiencies. Since methotrexate decreases appetite and it is, thus, contraindicated in patients with a poor nutritional status. The administration of cyclosporine along with grape fruit juice increases its oral bioavailability and can lead to toxicity. Patients on oral retinoids such as acitretin should be advised to avoid foods rich in vitamin A thus avoid hypervitaminosis.

Points to Remember

- Use low calorie diet
- Reduce weight
- Decrease/Stop acohol intake
- Increase the intake of PUFAs
- Increase the intake of fresh fruits and green leafy vegetables

REFERENCES

1. Kaimal S, Thappa DM. Diet in dermatology: Revisited. IJDVL. 2010;76(2):103-15.
2. Maurice PDL, Allen BR, Barkeley ASJ. The effects of dietary supplementation with fish oil in patients with psoriasis. Br J Dermatol. 1987;117(5):599-606.
3. Zackheim HS, Farber EM. Low protein diet and psoriasis. Arch Dermatol 1969;99(5):580-86.

Suggested Readings

1. Rook's Textbook of Dermatology.
2. Fitzpatrick's Dermatology in General Medicine.
3. IADVL Textbook of Dermatology.
4. Bolognia's Textbook of Dermatology.

Psoriasis at a Glance

- Psoriasis vulgaris is recognised as the most-prevalent autoimmune disease caused by inappropriate activation of the cellular immune system
- It is more common in whites and those who live farther from the equator and it is equally common in men and women
- Psoriasis is classified as a papulosquamous disorder. It occurs in 2–4% of the general population
- Psoriasis is more common with certain human leukocyte antigen (HLA) subtypes, e.g. HLA-CW6. Identification of susceptibility genes has pointed to a major role for both the innate and the adaptive immune system
- Psoriasis has a bimodal distribution of age of onset, the early or larger peak between 16 and 22 years and the later one at 57–60 years. The most common sites of involvement are the scalp, elbows and knees, followed by the nails, hands, feet and trunk
- Studies have shown that 30% of psoriasis patients have a first-degree relative with the condition
- Psoriasis is a complex autoimmune disease in which T cells are mistakenly activated, triggering other immune responses
- In India, the prevalence of psoriasis varies from 0.44 to 2.8%, it is twice more common in males compared to females and most of the patients are in their third or fourth decade at the time of presentation
- Children account for 4–5% of total psoriasis patients in India
- Genetic predisposition has a significant role in the etiopathogenesis of psoriasis and familial clustering of the cases has been observed
- There is a clear genetic contribution to psoriasis and psoriatic arthritis (PsA). Indian studies report lower familial incidence of the disease
- The presence of HLA-Cw*0602 is associated with more severe and early-onset psoriasis and has been found in approximately 100% of patients with guttate psoriasis
- Psoriasis is a chronic, immune-mediated disorder that results from a polygenic predisposition combined with environmental triggers, e.g. trauma, infections and medication
- Psoriasis is a multi-factorial skin disease with a complex pathogenesis
- Hyperproliferation of keratinocytes, T-cell activation, angiogenesis and cytokine mediators are believed to be involved in the pathogenesis of psoriasis
- Whether psoriasis represents a fundamental disease of skin, or the immune system has been debated for several years
- There are varied clinical presentations of psoriasis. Most common clinical type is the classic chronic plaque-type psoriasis. But even same clinical subtype can behave differently in different individuals
- It is important to recognize precisely the clinical subtype as it has implications on the choice of treatment modality and also reflects upon the disease activity
- Relapses are common and the patterns of relapses are also varied in different individuals. Some have early and frequent relapses and others have long-term remissions of their disease process with infrequent relapses
- Psoriasis has a number of clinical variants that differ in severity, location, longevity, shape, pattern, cause and treatment. The different types of psoriasis are fairly distinct. Patients may experience more than one type at the same time
- The prognosis is variable where there is preexisting, extensive-plaque psoriasis, treatment is usually well-tolerated and the prognosis is good; however, with unstable psoriasis, the course is often prolonged, relapses are frequent and there is an associated mortality

- Chronic-plaque psoriasis is the most common type
- Nail changes are observed in 25–50% of patients with psoriasis
- NAPSI is a numeric, reproducible, objective and simple tool for evaluation of nail psoriasis. This scale is used to evaluate the severity of nail-bed psoriasis and nail-matrix psoriasis by area of involvement in the nail unit
- Nail changes are more common in those with psoriatic arthritis and those with koebnerization
- Plaque psoriasis is the most common type of psoriasis
- Systemic retinoids are the treatment of first choice for generalized pustular psoriasis
- Systemic steroids are usually contraindicated in psoriasis except for the treatment of impetigo herpetiformis
- Psoriasis is associated with a high morbidity and a great level of psychological stress (Depression is more common)
- Metabolic syndrome, autoimmune diseases, parkinson's disease, hypertension, obesity, Type 2 diabetes and psoriatic arthritis is seen more commonly in patient's with psoriasis
- There are several associations of psoriasis including arthritis, immunobullous disorders, vitiligo, metabolic syndrome and synovitis, acne, pustulosis, hyperostosis and osteitis (SAPHO) syndrome. Arthritis is the most common association
- Metabolic syndrome has recently been found to be increasingly associated with psoriasis. Appropriate management of metabolic syndrome decreases the severity of psoriasis
- Psoriasis in children has few peculiar features which have been consistently observed in studies on childhood psoriasis. Guttate psoriasis is more common, spontaneous remissions are relatively more common than in adults while relapses usually follow infections. Certain clinical variants like erythroderma, localized and generalized pustular psoriasis and arthropathy are uncommon
- Western literature reports psoriasis prevalence to be around 0.71% in children
- Topical therapy remains the mainstay of treatment. Role of antibiotics remains controversial. Systemic therapies are used less often
- Management of psoriasis is a challenge and broadly consists of topical therapy, systemic therapy, physical and complimentary therapies and biological therapy
- Psoriasis covering less than 5% of BSA can be managed in most patients with the use of topical agents alone. These agents are the cornerstone of treatment for most patients with psoriasis
- Goeckerman therapy for psoriasis was first described at the Mayo Clinic in 1925 and is offered in various day-care clinics
- Acitretin, the active metabolite of etretinate, is the most commonly-used oral retinoid for psoriasis
- Acitretin as monotherapy is particularly considered to be effective in exfoliative erythrodermic psoriasis and pustular psoriasis. It has been extensively used in combination with ultraviolet B (UVB) or PUVA therapy for chronic plaque-type psoriasis
- Retinoids have several advantages over conventional systemic drugs like they are not immunosuppressive, there is no limitation of cumulative dose and they cause no significant hepatic or renal toxicity. Therefore, these are good candidates for combination and maintenance therapy both with conventional systemic anti-psoriatic drugs as well as with the biologic agents
- Cyclosporine (CSA) has the highest efficacy among all the nonbiologic systemic therapies. It is called the crisis drug as it is effective in cases resistant to other modalities and brings rapid control even in very-severe cases
- CSA cannot be used at the same time with psoralen + UVA (PUVA) or UVB phototherapy, methotrexate (MTX) or other immunosuppressive agents, coal tar, or radiation therapy
- CSA should be given in intermittent courses of maximum 12-weeks duration due to risk of renal damage. Another concern with CSA is the increased incidence of cutaneous squamous cell carcinomas

- MTX is a gold-standard drug in the management of psoriasis even in the era of biologicals
- The utility of folic acid (FA) supplementation with MTX use is debatable. Its use is advocated to limit the toxicity of MTX on liver, blood cells and gastrointestinal tract but there is a concern that it might reduce the efficacy of MTX
- MTX causes inhibition of 5-aminoimidazole-4-carboxamide ribonucleotide (AICAR) transformylase leading to accumulation of AICAR, which in turn causes increased tissue concentration of adenosine. Primarily, this increased tissue concentration of adenosine accounts for its anti-inflammatory properties leading to symptom alleviation in psoriasis
- Azathioprine is an immunosuppressant used in the treatment of blistering disorders, atopic dermatitis and various inflammatory dermatoses. There are no randomized trials but few open-label studies suggest its efficacy in psoriasis
- There is no FDA-approved use of azathioprine for psoriasis. Ideally TPMT levels should be done prior to the use of azathioprine
- There is no FDA approved use of fumarates in psoriasis. These are used in Northern Europe, particularly in Germany and Netherlands, as the first-line systemic treatment for moderate to severe psoriasis, with proven efficacy and low toxicity
- There is no FDA approved use of hydroxyurea in psoriasis
- Hydroxyurea is primarily used in the treatment of CML
- Hydroxyurea is a promising systemic treatment option for psoriasis because of less adverse effects
- Leflunomide, a pyrimidine synthesis inhibitor effective for rheumatoid arthritis, acts by inhibiting de novo pyrimidine synthesis. It is a disease-modifying antirheumatic drug which can be particularly beneficial for psoriasis patients with concurrent arthritis (PsA)
- MMF is a lymphocyte-selective immunosuppressive agent which acts by noncompetitive inhibition of de novo purine synthesis due to inhibition of inosine monophosphate dehydrogenase enzyme, thus resulting in blockade of T- and B-cell proliferation
- There is no FDA-approved use of MMF for psoriasis
- There is no FDA approved use of sulfasalazine in psoriasis. Currently it is FDA approved in the treatment of ulcerative colitis and rheumatoid arthritis
- Tacrolimus is rarely used for the treatment of psoriasis, but is a useful alternative
- Tacrolimus is not FDA approved for psoriasis
- 6-Thiogaunine is not FDA approved for the treatment of psoriasis. It is a useful alternative when other forms of treatment have failed
- Lupus vulgaris is the disease in which light therapy was first tried
- NBUVB has therapeutic efficacy equal to PUVA
- NBUVB is likely to be devoid of side-effects and will be considerably safe in the long-term than PUVA
- MED or MPD should be determined prior to the use of NBUVB and PUVA
- PUVA can be combined with retinoids, methotrexate, UVB and topical tazarotene
- The pregnancy category status of psoralens is C
- Calcipotriol should not be used concomitantly with phototherapy as it gets degraded by phototherapy
- Salicylic acid has photoprotective properties which will reduce the efficacy of phototherapy, hence should not be used concomitantly with phototherapy
- NBUVB phototherapy, is a potential advance in UVB-based phototherapy and is increasingly being used in the treatment of psoriasis. With regards to the relative therapeutic effectiveness of NB-UVB and PUVA, however, only sparse data are available. The mean cumulative clearance dose and adverse effects are lower in the NBUVB group than in the PUVA group
- Targeted phototherapy has been developed to treat localized disease (<10% body surface area) keeping the drawbacks of conventional phototherapy in mind

- NBUVB has been found to be a comparatively effective and relatively safer alternative to PUVA in more than two decades of use in the management of psoriasis
- Targeted NBUVB (dose applied at four-times MED) in combination with topical 0.1% 8-methoxypsoralen cream has been found to be much more efficacious in clearing psoriatic lesions compared with targeted phototherapy alone
- Most targeted phototherapy devices (laser or nonlaser type) emit radiation in the UVB range, with peak emission in the narrowband wavelength (around 308–311 nm)
- Targeted phototherapy may be achieved by different sources, such as excimer laser, IPL (excimer light) and UV light. The role of this modality both in diseases, such as vitiligo psoriasis and also in new indications such as acne and stretch marks continues to evolve
- Targeted phototherapy is devoid of the side effects of conventional phototherapy
- Biologicals are a recent addition to the therapeutic armamentarium of psoriasis. The biologics, because of their specific action on the immune system, have very little side effects
- The British Association of Dermatologists (2005) stated that candidates for biological therapies for psoriasis should have severe disease and fulfill at least one of the following criteria: Are or have become intolerant to or can not receive standard therapy, or are or have become unresponsive to standard therapy, or have developed or are at higher than average risk of developing clinically important drug-related toxicity and where alternative standard therapy can not be used, or have disease that is only controlled by repeated inpatient management, or have psoriatic arthritis fulfilling the British Society for Rheumatology (BSR) eligibility criteria for treatment with anti-tumor necrosis factor [TNF] agents, in association with skin disease, or have severe, unstable, life-threatening disease (erythrodermic or pustular psoriasis), or have significant, co-existant, unrelated co-morbidity that precludes the use of systemic agents, such as CSA or MTX.
- The use of complimentary therapies, such as climatotherapy, ichthyotherapy and balneotherapy should be considered in addition to the routine treatment to increase the duration of remission and improve the quality of life in patients with psoriasis
- Dietary interventions in psoriasis: Use low-calorie diet, reduce weight, decrease/stop acohol intake, increase the intake of PUFAs and fresh fruits and green-leafy vegetables.

Index

D

E

F

G

H

I

J

K

L

M

N

O

P

R

S

T

U

V

W

X